TECHNICAL
R E P O R T

Chronic Kidney Disease— A Quiet Revolution in Nephrology

Six Case Studies

Richard A. Rettig, Roberto B. Vargas, Keith C. Norris, Allen R. Nissenson

Sponsored by the National Institutes of Health, National Center for Research Resources

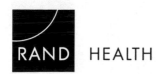

RAND HEALTH

This work was sponsored by the National Institutes of Health's National Center for Research Resources, which funded the Comprehensive Center for Health Disparities at Charles Drew University. The research was conducted in RAND Health, a division of the RAND Corporation.

Library of Congress Cataloging-in-Publication Data

Chronic kidney disease : a quiet revolution in nephrology : six case studies / Richard Rettig ... [et al.].
   p. ; cm.
   Includes bibliographical references.
   ISBN 978-0-8330-4972-8 (pbk. : alk. paper)
   1. Chronic renal failure--Treatment--United States--Case studies. 2. Outcome assessment (Medical care)--United States--Case studies. I. Rettig, Richard A. II. Rand Corporation.
  [DNLM: 1. Renal Insufficiency, Chronic--Practice Guideline. 2. Health Policy--Practice Guideline. 3. Outcome and Process Assessment (Health Care)--Practice Guideline. WJ 342 C5564 2010]

  RA645.K5C43 2010
  362.196'614--dc22

                   2010011740

The RAND Corporation is a nonprofit research organization providing objective analysis and effective solutions that address the challenges facing the public and private sectors around the world. RAND's publications do not necessarily reflect the opinions of its research clients and sponsors.

RAND® is a registered trademark.

Published 2010 by the RAND Corporation
1776 Main Street, P.O. Box 2138, Santa Monica, CA 90407-2138
1200 South Hayes Street, Arlington, VA 22202-5050
4570 Fifth Avenue, Suite 600, Pittsburgh, PA 15213-2665
RAND URL: http://www.rand.org/
To order RAND documents or to obtain additional information, contact
Distribution Services: Telephone: (310) 451-7002;
Fax: (310) 451-6915; Email: order@rand.org

Preface

Consistent with calls for reducing health disparities, in 2003 the Research Centers in Minority Institutions, part of the National Institutes of Health's (NIH's) National Center for Research Resources, funded the Comprehensive Center for Health Disparities (CCHD) at Charles Drew University of Science and Medicine (NIH/NCRR–RR019234) to address disparities in chronic kidney disease (CKD). The center is designed to take an integrated approach to the analysis and development of solutions to the burden of CKD and the disease's impact on society. Toward this aim, Charles Drew University, the David Geffen School of Medicine at the University of California at Los Angeles (UCLA), and the RAND Corporation partnered under the CCHD's Health Policy and Outcomes Core in conducting health services research and policy analyses aimed at identifying effective and efficient means to address prevention, early detection, and delivery of care for CKD at individual and community levels.

The confluence of several factors has created a unique opportunity in the study of CKD relevant to current and future health policy reform: (1) growing evidence of effective therapies for CKD prevention and care; (2) the increasing costs associated with end-stage renal disease (ESRD); and (3) the well-documented disparities in CKD outcomes and gaps in quality of care. This work represents the Health Policy and Outcomes Core's efforts toward providing policymakers, health administration leadership, and practicing clinicians with an in-depth descriptive analysis of the structural components, processes of care, and contextual factors that define the changing nature of the practice of care for patients with CKD in America. The findings from these real-world case studies offer policy-relevant examples and recommendations aimed at reducing the burden of CKD on the health system.

A profile of RAND Health, abstracts of its publications, and ordering information can be found at www.rand.org/health.

Contents

Preface iii
Figures ix
Tables xi
Summary xiii
Acknowledgments xvii
Abbreviations xix

CHAPTER ONE
Introduction: Chronic Kidney Disease, a Major Public Health Imperative 1
The Historical Context in Brief 2
Disparities 3
The Chronic Kidney Disease Guidelines 4
Barriers to Improved Patient Outcomes in Chronic Kidney Disease 6
Purpose of This Study and Methodological Approach 8
    The 2006 Telephone Survey 8
    The 2007 Case Studies 9
Organization of This Report 10

CHAPTER TWO
Overview of Findings 11
Findings from Telephone Interviews 11
Findings from Case Studies 12
Challenges for and Benefits of Chronic Kidney Disease Clinics and Practices 13
Conclusion 15

CHAPTER THREE
The Chronic Kidney Disease Clinic at Northwestern University, Chicago, Illinois 17
Practice Overview 17
Origins and Development of the Clinic 18
The Northwestern Chronic Kidney Disease Practice 20
    The Patient Population 20
    Outreach, Education, and Referrals 20
    Clinic Organization 21
    Clinic Procedures 21
    Practice Guidelines 22
    Treatment Outcomes 22

External Relations... 23
   Reimbursement 23
Future Challenges... 23

CHAPTER FOUR
Associates in Nephrology, Chicago, Illinois...25
Practice Overview..25
Origins and Development of the Clinic.. 26
The Associates in Nephrology Chronic Kidney Disease Practice 27
   The Patient Population 27
   Outreach, Education, and Referrals 28
   Clinic Organization 29
   Health Information Technology System 30
   Clinic Procedures 30
   Practice Guidelines 30
   Treatment Outcomes.. 30
External Relations..31
   Reimbursement 31
Future Challenges..31

CHAPTER FIVE
Mayo Clinic Nephrology, Jacksonville, Florida...33
Practice Overview..33
Origins and Development of the Clinic.. 34
The Mayo Clinic Chronic Kidney Disease Practice 34
   The Chronic Kidney Disease Clinic Patient Population 34
   Outreach, Education, and Referrals 36
   Clinic Procedures 37
   Health Information Technology System 38
   Practice Guidelines 39
External Relations..39
   Reimbursement 39
Future Challenges.. 40

CHAPTER SIX
Indiana Medical Associates, Fort Wayne, Indiana.. 41
Practice Overview.. 41
Origins and Development of Practice 42
The Indiana Medical Associates Chronic Kidney Disease Practice........................ 43
   The Patient Population 43
   Outreach, Education, and Referrals 43
   Practice Organization 44
   Health Information Technology Systems.. 44
   Clinic Procedures 44
   Practice Guidelines 45
External Relations.. 46

Reimbursement 46
Large Dialysis Organizations... 46

CHAPTER SEVEN

St. Clair Specialty Physicians, P.C., Detroit, Michigan 47
Practice Overview.. 47
Origins and Development 48
The St. Clair Chronic Kidney Disease Practice 48
    The Patient Population 49
    Outreach, Education, and Referrals 50
    Health Information Technology System 51
    Clinic Procedures 51
    Practice Guidelines 52
External Relations.. 52
    Reimbursement 52
Future Challenges.. 53

CHAPTER EIGHT

Winthrop University Hospital, Division of Nephrology and Hypertension, Mineola, Long Island, New York 55
Practice Overview.. 55
Origins and Development of Clinic 56
The Winthrop Chronic Kidney Disease Practice................................... 57
    The Patient Population 57
    Outreach, Education, and Referrals 57
    Clinic Organization 58
    Clinic Procedures 58
    Health Information Technology Systems 58
    Practice Guidelines 58
External Relations.. 59
    Reimbursement 59
Future Challenges.. 59

CHAPTER NINE

Conclusions and Recommendations 61
Conclusions.. 61
Policy Recommendations 62
Concluding Thoughts 65

APPENDIX

Interview Template 67

Endnotes.. 69

Figures

5.1. Mayo Clinic, Jacksonville, Chronic Kidney Disease Clinic Population 35
5.2. Distribution of Comorbidities Among Patients at the Mayo Clinic 36

Tables

1.1. Stages of Chronic Kidney Disease.. 5

1.2. Barriers Preventing Improved Patient Outcomes in Chronic Kidney Disease from the Chronic Kidney Disease Initiative, 2003 7

1.3. Clinics and Practices Participating in Case Studies 9

3.1. Healthy Living Clinic Chronic Kidney Disease Patients Compared with Doorstep End-Stage Renal Disease Patients... 19

4.1. Number of Chronic Kidney Disease Patients at the Associates in Nephrology Clinic, by Stage of Disease, October 2005–February 2006.. 27

4.2. Insurance Status of Chronic Kidney Disease Patients at the Associates in Nephrology Clinic, October 2005–February 2006.. 28

7.1. The St. Clair Patient Population, by Office (2000–2006) 49

Summary

For nearly 40 years, public policy has defined kidney disease primarily by its terminus—end-stage renal disease (ESRD). Recently, however, the disease entity of concern has been redefined as chronic kidney disease (CKD), a progressive disease that culminates in ESRD and that in most instances can be effectively treated in its earlier stages. Prevention is thus a possibility: Clinical interventions at earlier stages of CKD can effectively slow, stop, or, in some cases, reverse the progress to ESRD.

The possibility of preventing early-stage CKD from developing into kidney failure represents a still-unfolding area of innovation in nephrology. For medicine, CKD represents a challenge in moving from a chronic disease treatment model to a model that balances the relationship between prevention and care. For policy, the key issues involve the reimbursement of care, i.e., who will pay for the range of care associated with the expanded understanding of CKD.

There is a need for both practitioners and decisionmakers to better understand the CKD clinical practices capable of managing CKD throughout the disease continuum and of improving patient outcomes for kidney disease in the United States. This study represents an initial step in developing that understanding. Our Comprehensive Center for Health Disparities–Chronic Kidney Disease (CCHD–CKD) team, composed of researchers at Charles Drew University, the David Geffen School of Medicine at UCLA, and the RAND Corporation, has been conducting health services research within the CCHD's Health Policy and Outcomes Core, including this 2006–2007 study. The findings from this study offer descriptive examples of what leading nephrology practices around the United States are doing to address the challenges of CKD and provide the basis for a set of policy and clinical recommendations about how to advance the treatment of CKD.

A "Quiet Revolution" in Nephrology

In 1972, Congress extended Medicare entitlement to all individuals with a diagnosis of permanent kidney failure who needed dialysis or kidney transplantation to avoid death. This legislation led to a dramatic growth in the patient population, especially among the elderly, along with a corresponding rise in expenditures for treatment of the growing patient population. The increase in the patient population also revealed marked disparities in both the incidence and prevalence of ESRD among minority populations. The emergence of disparities did not represent a sudden increase in the number of cases of CKD among minorities; instead, the Medicare benefit gave providers an incentive to find and treat all patients, bringing many previously undiagnosed cases out into the open. In addition, Medicare began to document the changing demographics of the ESRD patient population, thus providing data that had previously been lacking.

Today, a quiet revolution is occurring in nephrology. The nature of the revolution was crystallized by the 2002 publication of the Kidney Disease Outcomes Quality Initiative (KDOQI) guidelines for the diagnosis and treatment of CKD, which described a progressive five-stage CKD model that incorporated ESRD as the final component of the overall model but provided direction for the early detection and treatment of CKD. Hence, the diagnosis of CKD has become relatively simple (for both nephrologists and non-nephrologists) through a process known as estimation of glomerular filtration rate (or eGFR), which, though not a direct measure of kidney function, estimates the ability of the kidneys to filter cellular toxins.

The framing of the disease as CKD shifts the focus from ESRD and represents a major change and innovation that is still unfolding. But this revolution has yet to receive adequate attention within nephrology and by policymakers, and some significant barriers remain to improved care for CKD patients.* Key among these is the fact that treatment for ESRD is paid for through Medicare, but early treatment of CKD is not. Other barriers include a lack of coordination between primary care physicians (PCPs) and nephrologists, a lack of public awareness regarding CKD, a lack of consensus among health care providers concerning the importance of CKD, and the need for data concerning the effectiveness of different tests and therapies for CKD.

Findings from Our Research

In 2006, we undertook a series of 15 telephone interviews, which were followed in 2007 by site visits to six CKD clinics or practices, to obtain an in-depth understanding of how diverse groups of leading nephrology practices around the United States are confronting the challenges of CKD. These findings offer descriptive examples of CKD practices and specific policy recommendations intended to improve patient outcomes for kidney disease in the United States.

Our telephone interviews raised several key themes concerning CKD practices today, many of which were later echoed in the case studies. Most practices we interviewed favored early intervention, although several expressed ambivalence, and a few thought the payoff was greater when treatments were started in later stages of CKD. The practices identified a number of problems and challenges in treating CKD patients, including limited reimbursement, lack of patient awareness of CKD, and difficulty in identifying CKD patients and in creating patient histories from multiple sources. Relations between nephrologists and other medical specialists—PCPs (internists, family practitioners), cardiologists, and endocrinologists— elicited a good deal of comment. In general, nephrologists felt that patients were being referred for CKD care too late, although respondents also noted a recent trend toward earlier referrals. The practices we interviewed organized CKD care in a variety of ways: Some lacked any formal approach to CKD care, others emphasized CKD but lacked a clear organization, and others had established clinics specifically focused on CKD.

---

*   In February 2003, the Council of American Kidney Societies (CAKS) identified 19 barriers to improved patient outcomes in CKD, including specific aspects of both the delivery and financing of care for CKD.

The case studies provide details about these findings and shed light in particular on several of the challenges faced by CKD clinics, as well as some of the ways in which clinics are addressing these challenges. Specifically, these findings include:

Reimbursement. The major barrier to clinic operations involved limitations on reimbursement of CKD. All six of the CKD clinics and practices in the case studies face financial challenges in providing CKD care, especially to support the multidisciplinary staff of nurses and other health professionals needed for a comprehensive practice.

Patient Referral. All CKD clinics and practices in the study have confronted the need to reach out to PCPs, cardiologists, and endocrinologists to ensure the predictable referral of patients for CKD care before patients need immediate dialysis. There was concern among nephrologists that PCPs were reluctant to refer for fear of losing patients, but this concern was tempered in academic and integrated CKD clinics by targeted efforts to comanage CKD with PCPs.

Patient Screening. The ability to screen potential CKD patients varied across clinics but was generally limited by weak referral patterns in nonintegrated health systems and limited public awareness of the need for early-stage care. The use of eGFR and community outreach programs was cited as a factor in increasing early-stage referrals.

Patient and Provider Education. The need to educate both patients and PCPs was seen as critical, both to increase patient awareness of CKD and to ensure that physicians know the early indications of CKD. All CKD clinics engaged in some educational efforts, including presentations, public service announcements, and provider education.

Practice Organization. Clinic organization remains quite varied and in flux. The structures of the clinics in our case studies varied greatly. Some nephrology divisions of large multi-specialty group practices had carved out a CKD clinic within that context, while in others the CKD effort was an extension of a clinical base in ESRD.

Use of Clinical Practice Guidelines. Guidance is increasingly available through continuously updated clinical practice guidelines (CPGs). All CKD clinics in our study used CPGs as a first-order means to identify patients, organize practices, and build data systems. All of the clinics visited adapted the guidelines for local and patient-specific purposes.

Health Information Technology. The use of health information technology (HIT) can facilitate CKD care. The six CKD clinics varied greatly in the stage of development of their HIT systems. Some have purchased off-the-shelf products, while others have developed their own. One site received financial assistance from a state and federal government effort to encourage the transition to electronic medical records.

CKD Disparities. Unfortunately, the racial and ethnic disparities prevalent in the ESRD population appear also in the CKD population, but, without reimbursement, referral patterns and levels of patient knowledge often go undetected. In our case studies, sites that served predominantly minority and underserved communities had patients presenting at much younger ages and with more advanced disease. In response, they employed targeted community outreach and educational programs.

The case studies also highlighted a number of benefits that flow from CKD clinics, including the advantages of early treatment, success in using the estimation of GFR for early referrals, and the increasing possibility of preemptive kidney transplantation.

Policy Recommendations

On the basis of the telephone interviews and the six case studies, we developed a set of policy and clinical recommendations about how to advance the treatment of chronic kidney disease. The following set of recommendations provides a blueprint for reengineering CKD in the United States:

- Appropriate reimbursement needs to be available to screen at-risk populations and to enable ongoing care by physicians as CKD is diagnosed and progresses.
- Patient referral, the other critical resource, requires negotiations between nephrologists and other providers and specialists at the local clinic or practice level, as well as at the level of the pertinent professional societies.
- Screening patients for CKD by eGFR should be made obligatory by Medicare and state Medicaid agencies, and private insurers should be strongly encouraged to pay for such screening.
- Education is critical. Both patients and providers need to be educated about the prevalence of CKD, who is at risk, who should be treated, and which treatments are effective in slowing the progression of the disease, as well as treating its complications and those associated with comorbid conditions that are present.
- CKD clinical practice needs to integrate the efforts of PCPs, cardiologists, endocrinologists, nephrologists, and nonphysician care providers to optimize clinical outcomes. Coordinated care management, relying on available best medical evidence, needs to drive clinical decisions and practice.
- Available clinical practice guidelines, such as the Kidney Disease Outcomes Quality Initiative (KDOQI) guidelines published by the National Kidney Foundation (NKF) and the Renal Physicians Association (RPA) guidelines, need to be integrated into actual clinical practice.
- Consistent with current health reform efforts, robust HIT is essential to track and evaluate care across various delivery sites.
- Nephrologists and other providers need to be held accountable for the outcomes of their patients.
- Substantial investments in translational and health services research are needed to better understand how to prevent CKD, treat it when it occurs, and carry out these activities efficiently and effectively.

The crisis of nephrology lies in an unresolved tension between the specialty's increasing ability to do the right thing clinically (by providing effective preventive care) and the persistent realities of major barriers to doing so, including inadequate reimbursement, weak working relations between nephrology and other specialties, organizational impediments, ineffective clinical procedures, and a lack of HIT systems. To the extent that our observations identify models of improved access to CKD care for all individuals as well as efforts targeted at minority populations, this work may help eliminate disparities in kidney disease outcomes. Action on CKD policy will equip clinicians with the basic tools to respond to such factors.

Acknowledgments

We thank the principals of the six CKD clinics and practices described in this report who graciously provided information in site visit interviews and later reviewed their respective chapters for accuracy. They are Daniel Batlle, M.D., Cybele Ghossein, M.D., and James Paparello, M.D., of Northwestern University, Chicago, Illinois; Paul W. Crawford, M.D., of Associates in Nephrology, Chicago, Illinois; Robert Provenzano, M.D., of St. Clair Specialty Physicians, P.C., Detroit, Michigan; Stephen McMurray, M.D., of Indiana Medical Associates, Fort Wayne, Indiana; William Haley, M.D., Peter Fitzpatrick, M.D., and James Dwyer, M.D., of the Mayo Clinic, Jacksonville, Florida; and Stephen Fishbane, M.D., of Winthrop University Hospital, Mineola, New York. We thank these individuals and their staffs for their help in this report and for the pioneering clinical work they are performing in providing chronic kidney disease care. Consequently, we have listed the principals of these clinics and practices as coauthors of their respective cases.

We also wish to thank our reviewers for their helpful input: Alan Kliger, M.D., of Yale University; John Sadler, M.D., of Independent Dialysis Foundation, Baltimore, Maryland; and Hank Green, Ph.D., of RAND.

Abbreviations

ACE	angiotensin-converting enzyme
AHA	American Heart Association
AIN	Associates in Nephrology
APN	advanced practice nurse
ARB	angiotensin II receptor blocker
AV	arteriovenous
CAKS	Council of American Kidney Societies
CCHD	Comprehensive Center for Health Disparities
CCHD–CKD	Comprehensive Center for Health Disparities–Chronic Kidney Disease
CKD	chronic kidney disease
CKDI	Chronic Kidney Disease Initiative
CMS	Centers for Medicare and Medicaid Services
CPG	clinical practice guideline
CV	cardiovascular
eGFR	estimated glomerular filtration rate
EHR	electronic health record
EMR	electronic medical record
EPO	erythropoietin
ESRD	end-stage renal disease
FMC	Fresenius Medical Care
GFR	glomerular filtration rate
HIT	health information technology
HLC	Healthy Living Clinic

IMA	Indiana Medical Associates
KDOQI	Kidney Disease Outcomes Quality Initiative
LPN	licensed practical nurse
MDRD	Modification of Diet in Renal Disease
NIH	National Institutes of Health
NKF	National Kidney Foundation
NP	nurse practitioner
PA	physician assistant
PCP	primary care physician
RCG	Renal Care Group
RN	registered nurse
RPA	Renal Physicians Association
UCLA	University of California at Los Angeles
USRDS	U.S. Renal Data System

CHAPTER ONE

Introduction: Chronic Kidney Disease, a Major Public Health Imperative

Richard A. Rettig, Ph.D.; Keith C. Norris, M.D.; Allen R. Nissenson, M.D.;
Roberto B. Vargas, M.D., M.P.H.

For nearly 40 years, public policy has defined kidney disease primarily by its terminus, end-stage renal disease (ESRD). Treatment for those diagnosed with kidney failure has typically focused on dialysis or kidney transplantation, the effectiveness of which was demonstrated by the 1960s. The Social Security Amendments of 1972 established a Medicare entitlement for those with a diagnosis of kidney failure who required treatment by dialysis or kidney transplantation. At that time, no strategies to prevent ESRD existed.

While ESRD is still the main focus of kidney disease–related care today, in recent years more attention has been given to treating all stages of chronic kidney disease (CKD), including those preceding ESRD. In 2002, the Kidney Disease Outcomes Quality Initiative (KDOQI) of the National Kidney Foundation (NKF) published guidelines for diagnosing and treating CKD.[1] These guidelines redefined the disease as a five-stage progressive condition that included ESRD as the final stage. Prevention is now a possibility: Clinical interventions at earlier stages of CKD can effectively slow, stop, or in some cases reverse the progress to ESRD. This development means that nephrology is no longer exclusively focused on ESRD, even though the bulk of the specialty remains occupied with dialysis and kidney transplantation. The possibility of preventing early-stage CKD from developing into kidney failure represents a still-unfolding area of innovation in nephrology, and effective treatments for earlier stages of CKD are still emerging. Thus, there is a need for practitioners as well as decisionmakers to better understand the CKD clinical practices capable of managing CKD throughout the disease continuum and of improving patient outcomes for kidney disease in the United States.

In addition, the growing emphasis on CKD rather than ESRD alone has posed epidemiological challenges. The redefinition of CKD as a five-stage disease means that the population at risk has grown dramatically since the 1970s, especially among the elderly. The number of individuals with some stage of CKD is estimated to be nearly 30 million,[2] and having CKD is becoming recognized as an important risk factor for premature mortality.[3, 4] Of the total CKD population, each year nearly 500,000 individuals with ESRD are treated with renal replacement therapy (dialysis and kidney transplantation) at a cost of about $35 billion.[5] Disparities in the incidence and prevalence of ESRD among African-Americans and other minorities represent another CKD-related public health challenge.

Moreover, in financial terms, the need to differentiate CKD care from that for ESRD has also become a significant policy issue. It is now clinically possible to intervene effectively at earlier stages of CKD, and, in doing so, the financial burden of ESRD care can be reduced. However, these savings are offset to some extent by the increased patient population being treated. The number of prospective CKD patients in earlier stages is substantially higher than the number of patients at stage 5 (ESRD). In addition, ESRD treatment is paid for through Medicare, while, in general, CKD care for earlier stages is not.

This study attempts to provide insights into the current state of CKD care by examining the efforts of several leading CKD clinics and practices that have been established in recent years. In 2006, our Comprehensive Center for Health Disparities–Chronic Kidney Disease (CCHD–CKD) team, composed of researchers at Charles Drew University, the RAND Corporation, and the David Geffen School of Medicine at the University of California, Los Angeles, conducted telephone interviews with 15 CKD practices and, in 2007, carried out on-site case studies with six practices. The case study approach was adopted to generate detailed descriptive data about CKD care that could not be obtained through quantitative methods. The case studies demonstrate the challenges associated with CKD care, illustrate several models of CKD care being used to address these challenges, and establish the basis for policy recommendations for advancing the treatment of CKD.

In the remainder of this introduction, we provide a brief discussion of the historical context for understanding CKD, including racial and ethnic disparities in disease prevalence and treatment, current guidelines for CKD care, and barriers to improved patient outcomes. We also describe our study focus in more detail, as well as the approach used in the interviews and case studies.

The Historical Context in Brief

In 1972, Congress extended Medicare entitlement, originally established for the elderly in 1965, to two previously uncovered groups of all ages: the disabled and those individuals with a diagnosis of permanent kidney failure who needed dialysis or kidney transplantation to avoid death. This legislation came long after the first artificial kidney machine was developed in the mid-1940s, long after treatment of chronic kidney failure became possible, and a decade after the federal government began to respond to these life-saving clinical innovations through the Veterans Administration, the Public Health Service, and the National Institutes of Health (NIH). Congressional action also resolved a decade of sustained ethical controversy over access to dialysis, which was frequently rationed because of limited government reimbursement for treatment.

The 1972 legislation had three major effects. First, there was a dramatic growth in the patient population, especially among the elderly. In 1973–1974, the first full year of the program, the number of Medicare beneficiaries of all ages receiving ESRD therapy was approximately 10,000. That number grew steadily to 59,962 by 1980, 186,493 by 1990, 392,140 by 2000, and to 506,256 by the end of 2006. Diabetes, once a contraindication for treatment, also emerged as a major contributor of renal failure.

Second, a relentless rise in expenditures for treatment occurred. In 2006, Medicare expenditures for ESRD services reached $23 billion, or 6.4 percent of total Medicare expenditures.[6] Total costs reflect both the aging and increasing complexity of the population being treated. Less than 20 percent of the costs go toward dialysis treatment, while another 22 percent represent the cost of injectable medications (erythropoietin [EPO], iron, vitamin D), and nearly 40 percent go toward hospitalization.[7]

The third effect of the 1972 legislation was the emergence of marked disparities in both the incidence and prevalence of ESRD among minority populations, especially African-Americans, but also Hispanics and Asian Americans. Before the 1972 legislation, there was little indication that black-white disparities would be as dramatic as they later became. The National Dialysis Registry,* the primary source of dialysis data before 1972, classified patients by age and sex but provided no data on race.[8] The Human Renal Transplant Registry† collected ethnicity data but had found no significant disparities: For the years of 1971 through 1974, African-American recipients of kidney transplants constituted 9.2, 9.8, 11.3, and 11.9 percent, respectively, of all recipients. These results were not at all disproportionate to the proportion of African-Americans in the general population.[9] However, once the near-universal Medicare benefit was implemented, racial and ethnic disparities emerged more clearly and became a reality for American nephrologists.

The emergence of disparities in the incidence and prevalence of ESRD did not represent a sudden increase in the number of cases of ESRD among minorities, but the recognition of disparities that already existed. The Medicare benefit gave providers an incentive to find and treat all patients, thus bringing many previously undiagnosed cases into the open. In addition, Medicare began to document the changing demographics of the ESRD patient population, especially from the 1980s onward through the U.S. Renal Data System (USRDS), in collaboration with the NIH, thus providing data that had previously been lacking.

As the number of diagnosed cases increased, racial and ethnic disparities among ESRD patients became apparent.[10, 11] In the most recent report of the USRDS (2008), for example, the rates of new ESRD patients among African-Americans and Native Americans were 3.6 and 1.8 times greater, respectively, than that for whites; the incidence for Hispanics was 1.5 times that for non-Hispanics; and African-American recipients of kidney transplants constituted 8.5, 8.6, and 8.0 percent of all transplants in 2004–2006.[12, 13] These rate differentials resulted from disparities in ESRD prevalence and incidence: In 2006, African-American patients accounted, respectively, for 31.6 percent of the prevalent ESRD population and 28.2 percent of the incident population; Native Americans accounted for 1.3 percent of the prevalent population and 1 percent of incident patients; and Hispanics constituted 14.3 percent and 13.2 percent of prevalent and incident patients, respectively.[14]

Disparities

CKD illustrates one of the most common burdens associated with inadequate health care in the United States: the overrepresentation of underserved and minority individuals suffering from chronic illness. In the United States, there remain marked differences in health outcomes by sociocultural, racial/ethnic, and geographic stratifications.[15, 16] In his 2007 Shattuck Lecture, Dr. Steven A. Schroeder underlined this point: "Since all the actionable determinants of health—personal behavior, social factors, health care, and the environment—disproportionately affect the poor, strategies to improve national health rankings must focus on this popu-

---

* The National Dialysis Registry was developed and maintained by the Research Triangle Institute under contract to the National Institute of Arthritis and Metabolic Diseases and issued annual reports from 1967 through 1978.

† The Human Renal Transplant Registry was developed and maintained by the American College of Surgeons under contract to the National Institute of Allergy and Infectious Diseases and issued annual reports from 1964 through 1977.

lation."[17] Many health care leaders support efforts to reduce health disparities and are seeking to identify effective clinical interventions to support needed policy changes.[18, 19, 20, 21] The CCHD–CKD, the NIH-funded entity carrying out this project, is an example of such efforts charged with conducting research to reduce disparities in access to and quality of CKD care for vulnerable populations.

The observed racial and ethnic differences in the epidemiology of kidney disease arise out of the complex relationship among biological, sociodemographic, and behavioral factors.[22] These factors often lead to tension in the selection of policies to reduce ethnic and racial disparities. Studies have produced mixed findings concerning the effectiveness of various interventions. Some studies have shown that population-based quality improvement efforts in the Medicare ESRD population reduce racial and gender disparities in quality of care.[23] However, other studies have demonstrated that racial and ethnic disparities in treatment persist (e.g., nephrologists are more or less likely to refer patients for transplantation depending on the patient's race or ethnicity) even after adjusting for sociodemographic, clinical, and patient preference differences for kidney transplantation.[24]

The Chronic Kidney Disease Guidelines

Today, a quiet revolution is occurring in nephrology—characterized by a shift from treating only ESRD to managing CKD throughout the spectrum of the disease. But this revolution has yet to receive adequate attention within nephrology and by policymakers. The nature of the revolution was crystallized by the 2002 publication of the National Kidney Foundation's KDOQI guidelines for the diagnosis and treatment of CKD.[25] These NKF guidelines, and similar guidelines developed by the Renal Physicians Association (RPA), are the products of an ongoing and now deep-rooted practice within nephrology of developing clinical practice guidelines, which has been on the whole a beneficial process, though not one without controversy.[26]

The NKF CKD guidelines‡ include multiple components:

- definition and classification of CKD in five progressive stages, with ESRD as the final stage
- evaluation of laboratory measurements for assessing kidney disease, specifically, the estimation of residual renal function
- association of residual renal function with hypertension, anemia, nutrition, bone disease, neuropathy, and patient well-being
- stratification of the risk of progression of CKD to ESRD and to the development of cardiovascular disease
- recommendations for clinical performance measures and use of the guidelines.

In the five-stage CKD model, the guidelines define kidney disease in terms of kidney function rather than disease type (see Table 1.1). Each stage of CKD is defined by a marker of kidney damage (e.g., proteinuria) or a decrease of kidney function that persists for three or more months. Each stage is also associated with an estimate of glomerular filtration rate (eGFR) shown in the right column of Table 1.1, which, though not a direct measure of kidney

---

‡   There are 15 guidelines in the 2002 document.

Table 1.1
Stages of Chronic Kidney Disease

Stage	Description	eGFR (mL/min./1.73 m2)
1	Kidney damage with normal or increased eGFR	>90
2	Kidney damage with mildly decreased eGFR	60–89
3	Moderately decreased eGFR	30–59
4	Severely decreased eGFR	15–29
5	Kidney failure	<15 (or dialysis)

NOTE: Table adapted from NKF, KDOQI Clinical Practice Guidelines for CKD, *Am J Kid Dis*, 2002;39(Suppl 1):S46.

function, estimates the ability of the kidneys to filter cellular toxins (measured through a blood test). Stages 2 through 5 represent a progressively declining value in the filtering ability of the kidney. When the eGFR is 100, the kidneys are filtering at the normal level. An eGFR of 50 reflects a level of kidney function that is about one-half of normal, and an eGFR of 33 reflects a level of kidney function that is about one-third of normal. Patients with stage 1 CKD have fairly well-preserved filtering ability (eGFR greater than 90), but there is other evidence of early kidney damage, such as persistent proteinuria, which can be detected in patients using a simple urine-screening test.

The definition of CKD and its stages represents the culmination of various strands of clinical research and treatment that have emphasized the need for early clinical evaluation and preparation for dialysis. For many years there have been reports of patients "crashing" at a nephrologist's doorstep in the final stage of kidney failure, never having seen a nephrologist previously but now needing immediate dialysis. Such "doorstep patients" drew attention to the need for prior clinical evaluation and preparation for dialysis, especially in the creation of an arteriovenous (AV) fistula to provide vascular access.[27, 28] In the late 1990s, the Centers for Medicare and Medicaid Services (CMS) launched a national initiative known as Fistula First to increase the use of fistulas among patients before the immediate need for dialysis. This initiative emerged from the recognition that it is important to adequately prepare patients for hemodialysis.[29, 30] Another important clinical advance has focused on slowing the progression of CKD through blood pressure control by use of medications such as angiotensin-converting enzyme (ACE) inhibitors and angiotensin II receptor blockers (ARBs).[31, 32] Blood sugar control has also been extremely important, as diabetes is a major CKD risk factor and a major contributor to ESRD.[33]

The CKD guidelines highlighted the need for standardized criteria and procedures of patient referral to assist the relationship between primary care physicians (PCPs) and nephrologists. The estimation of glomerular filtration rate (GFR) was intended to make the diagnosis of CKD relatively simple, both for nephrologists and non-nephrologists (e.g., PCPs, cardiologists, and endocrinologists) and to facilitate the early identification and appropriate treatment of CKD, which is largely asymptomatic in early stages. Dr. Andrew Levey, who chaired the NKF group that developed the CKD guidelines, put it this way: "We developed an equation to estimate GFR. . . . the equation was not used until we defined CKD, a definition based on GFR. But [GFR] gave every internist a tool, a definition, something to do."[34]

Although the use of staging has helped PCPs to identify CKD, the guideline also has the potential to create unintended consequences. For example, some physicians may believe that guideline-based staging alone is sufficient to diagnose CKD. The result may be that the physician simply assumes that hypertension or diabetes has caused CKD in a patient, while missing the early opportunity for a thorough renal evaluation leading to definitive diagnosis and potentially early disease-specific therapy.

Further, although the eGFR remains the clinical standard, it is limited by variability across age and select patient populations. For example, the use of a single eGFR remains less well defined for classifying stage 1 or 2 CKD compared with stages 3–5, since most of the data for the formula were generated for patients with stages 3–5. Moreover, staging may lead some elderly patients to be labeled as having CKD (because of a reduced eGFR) when they are not at risk for CKD progression or complications.

The limitations of the eGFR underscore its role as a tool, not a marker of definitive diagnosis. Premature diagnosis can lead to patient anxiety and unnecessary tests and treatments without a more comprehensive clinical approach. Further studies are needed to move from staging based on expert opinion toward staging based on validated evidence that can provide better guidance about when nephrology input is needed and when it may be delayed.

These difficulties notwithstanding, the staging delineated by the CKD guidelines and the reliance on eGFR for determination of stage constitute major clinical advances over the pre-guideline period. The staging provides a framework for organizing appropriate interventions for clinicians while also permitting clearer evaluation of published evidence regarding pathophysiology, treatment, and prevention of CKD and its complications. The simplified staging framework can also serve as a platform to facilitate patient awareness and education about the risk of disease and prevention of disease progression.

Barriers to Improved Patient Outcomes in Chronic Kidney Disease

Notwithstanding the progress that has resulted from the guidelines, some significant barriers remain to improved care for CKD patients. In February 2003, the Council of American Kidney Societies (CAKS) met to discuss the implications of the prior year's KDOQI guidelines.[35] Forty-eight individuals, including the authors of this study, participated in this effort—among them nephrologists, PCPs, nurses, physician extenders, payers, epidemiologists, academicians, and representatives of government agencies, dialysis provider organizations, disease management organizations, and professional nephrology societies. The CAKS discussions identified 19 barriers to improved patient outcomes in CKD (see the left column of Table 1.2), which were summarized in the Chronic Kidney Disease Initiative (CKDI).[36] Specific aspects of both the delivery and financing of care for CKD were highlighted as prominent barriers to advancing care for this vulnerable population.

Most of the barriers to care remain unresolved today. The right column in Table 1.2 shows our team's evaluation of the progress made in nephrology in addressing the barriers to CKD care since the CAKS meeting in 2003. This evaluation was based, in part, on findings from the interviews and case studies as well as on our team's expertise, involvement, and knowledge of nephrology literature and federal government policy. The team concluded that,

Table 1.2
Barriers Preventing Improved Patient Outcomes in Chronic Kidney Disease from the Chronic Kidney Disease Initiative, 2003

CKDI Appraisal (2003)	CCHD–CKD Appraisal (2007–2008)
1. eGFR not reported by laboratories	Lab reporting of eGFR is slowly increasing and is now estimated at 40 percent.
2. Lack of public and patient awareness and concern regarding the risks associated with CKD	Increased outreach activities are occurring, but uptake remains slow.
3. Maldistribution and worsening shortage of health care providers	The shortage of providers is not getting better, and is probably getting worse.
4. Lack of coordination between PCPs and nephrologists	There is some evidence of improvement, but more efforts are needed.
5. Unwillingness among payers to cover and reimburse early CKD care	This key issue has not been resolved.
6. Need for payers to recognize the value of early treatment of CKD	This key issue also remains unresolved.
7. Absence of a coordinated system of care that includes a delivery system that will reach all CKD patients	A coordinated system remains an ideal to be sought in the next decade.
8. Inadequate recognition that ESRD is not the only patient outcome of CKD, which can also lead to cardiovascular disease and complications of decreased GFR	This is a vital clinical issue, both for nephrologists and other specialties. Increased educational activities are occurring, but uptake remains slow.
9. CKD conceptualization is very recent and not widely diffused within nephrology, medicine, or the health care system.	This conceptualization has been and remains a fundamental limiting factor.
10. Lack of consensus regarding the importance of CKD	There has been some progress, but there remains a need for joint statements on CKD among nephrology, cardiology, endocrinology, general internal medicine, and family practice specialty organizations.
11. Need for data on variations in care process, outcomes, and best practices	The CKD care structure needs to be enhanced to allow for systematic data collection.
12. Lack of consensus on how the marketing of CKD message should be structured and implemented	Various marketing models exist—capture model, evangelism model, entrepreneurial model—but none has yet emerged as dominant.
13. Inadequate understanding of optimal context for CKD screening, prevention, and treatment	A need exists to better connect the structure and processes of nephrology/CKD practices and primary care practices, ideally through a CKD clinic.
14. Need for nephrology leadership to unite and speak with a single voice on this issue	There may be a need for a convening authority, perhaps a study by the Institute of Medicine.
15. Lack of convincing cost-benefit data	This constitutes a critical economic issue. More effective and comprehensive cost-benefit modeling is needed.
16. Lack of acceptance of a uniform definition of CKD	This technical issue has been largely resolved by the KDOQI guidelines.
17. Lack of understanding about those CKD patients most likely to benefit from interventions	This issue highlights the need to understand which CKD diagnoses are most amenable to evidenced-based interventions.
18. Risk that no entity exists with a broad mandate to sustain these efforts over the long term	Currently, no payer—CMS/Medicare, state Medicaid programs, or private insurers—is adequately paying for CKD care.

Table 1.2—Continued

CKDI Appraisal (2003)	CCHD–CKD Appraisal (2007–2008)
19. Lack of prospective evidence for effective tests and therapies to prevent complications of CKD	A growing body of evidence supports early intervention with positive results. The opportunity exists for observational studies with clinical data; financing for intervention trials is limited.

NOTE: Adapted from CKDI,[37] with permission.

although nephrologists are now devoting more time to managing CKD patients, key issues remain, including a lack of coordination between PCPs and nephrologists, problems with reimbursement for early CKD care, a lack of public awareness regarding CKD, a lack of consensus among health care providers concerning the importance of CKD, and the need for evidence concerning the effectiveness of different tests and therapies for CKD.

Purpose of This Study and Methodological Approach

The barriers to CKD highlighted above underscore the need for policies and clinical practices that lead to improved outcomes for CKD patients, especially those in the early stages of the disease. In particular, our evaluation of progress in addressing the barriers identified by the CKDI of 2003 (Table 1.2) pointed to many continuing challenges. This evaluation served as a guide for a 2006 telephone survey with CKD practitioners and a series of 2007 site visits to CKD clinics and practices. Our research team sought to understand clinicians' views on such topics as early intervention for CKD, challenges in treating CKD patients, relationships between nephrology practices and other medical specialties, and the organization and reimbursement of CKD care.

The study was also motivated by the authors' own long-term involvement in ESRD and CKD. Drs. Nissenson and Norris, both nephrologists, have each been engaged in both clinical practice and CKD-related clinical research for several decades. Dr. Nissenson served in 1999–2001 as president of the RPA and as a longtime board member. Dr. Norris, also a former RPA board member, has conducted NIH-funded research on kidney disease and various aspects of health disparities for many years. Dr. Rettig, as a social scientist, has written extensively about ESRD and directed the Institute of Medicine study that resulted in *Kidney Failure and the Federal Government* in 1991.[38] Dr. Vargas, co-leader of the Health Policy and Outcomes core of the CCHD–CKD, is an internist and health services researcher with expertise in the description and analysis of health care interventions and the use of community engagement in raising awareness of CKD.[39, 40, 41]

The 2006 Telephone Survey
At the time of the CAKS meeting and until the 2008 Annual Data Report of the USRDS, very little systematic data existed on CKD care at the clinic or practice level. In 2006, therefore, we undertook a series of telephone interviews with 14 nephrologists and one staff member (the latter from RPA) in order to provide a qualitative understanding of what was occurring at the

level of CKD clinical practice.§ The research team members identified potential interviewees during a telephone conference.

All interviews were scheduled and conducted by Dr. Rettig using a semistructured interview instrument developed in consultation with the other team members. The interview template used is provided in the appendix. Dr. Rettig summarized his interview notes, which were returned in draft form to the interviewee for review and comment. Dr. Rettig then prepared final notes for each interview and a summary of all interviews. Dr. Rettig and the team reviewed the results from the interviews and identified key themes, which were shared with the interviewees. These themes are described in Chapter Two of this report.

The 2007 Case Studies

Guided by the themes from the telephone interviews, we initiated case studies of six CKD clinics and practices known to be engaged in CKD care. The purpose of the case studies was to obtain an in-depth qualitative understanding of how leading nephrology practices around the United States were confronting the challenges of CKD care. Case study clinics and practices were chosen for their illustrative purposes, not as a representative sample. Indeed, we were quite conscious that the great majority of ESRD centers are not yet engaged in CKD care. The sites were drawn from among those practices that participated in the telephone interviews. Participating clinics and practices are shown in Table 1.3.

Dr. Rettig scheduled and conducted all site visit interviews, which involved the clinic director at all sites, as well as other participating physicians at two sites. Each semistructured interview lasted between one and one-half and two hours. Dr. Rettig wrote up interview notes immediately after each site visit and provided the notes to interviewees for review for accuracy; follow-up phone calls augmented interview data when needed. Interviewees also provided published papers, poster presentations, and other materials pertaining to their clinic. The final write-up for each clinic or practice, prepared by Dr. Rettig, was reviewed by the CCHD–CKD research team, all of whom contributed to the writing of this report.

These case studies describe the realities of CKD care in ways relevant to members of Congress and other policymakers. The issues surrounding CKD cannot be resolved within

Table 1.3
Clinics and Practices Participating in Case Studies

Clinic or Practice	Leadership
CKD Clinic at Northwestern University, Chicago, Ill.	Daniel Batlle, M.D.
Associates in Nephrology (AIN) Chronic Kidney Disease Clinic, Chicago, Ill.	Paul W. Crawford, M.D.
Mayo Clinic Nephrology, Jacksonville, Fla.	William E. Haley, M.D.
Indiana Medical Associates, Fort Wayne, Ind.	Stephen McMurray, M.D.
St. Clair Specialty Physicians, P.C., Detroit, Mich.	Robert Provenzano, M.D.
Winthrop University Hospital, Division of Nephrology and Hypertension, Long Island, N.Y.	Stephen Fishbane, M.D.

§ The interviewees were Drs. Daniel Batlle, Chaim Charytan, Paul Crawford, Stephen Fishbane, William Haley, Alan Kliger, Jill Lindberg, Stephen McMurray, Lionel Mailloux, Robert Provenzano, John Sadler, Ajay Singh, Theodore Steinman, and James Weiss.

nephrology alone but require conscious policy action, especially to ensure that health care providers are reimbursed for their services to CKD patients, which is essential if clinical improvements are to develop further. Findings from the case studies are summarized in Chapter Two, with findings for individual practices discussed in Chapters Three through Eight. Chapter Nine discusses our policy and clinical recommendations.

In 2008, we are pleased to note, the USRDS devoted a complete volume to CKD in its 2008 Annual Data Report; it did so again in its 2009 Annual Data Report and will do so annually. In our view, aggregate data and case study data are complementary and enhance understanding of developments with respect to CKD care.

Organization of This Report

The remainder of this report presents the findings and recommendations from our study:

- Chapter Two provides an overview of the key findings from both the telephone interviews and the case studies.
- Chapters Three through Eight provide detailed discussions of the six clinics and practices participating in the case studies:
  - Chapter Three: The CKD Clinic at Northwestern University, Chicago, Illinois
  - Chapter Four: Associates in Nephrology (AIN) Chronic Kidney Disease Clinic, Chicago, Illinois
  - Chapter Five: Mayo Clinic Nephrology, Jacksonville, Florida
  - Chapter Six: Indiana Medical Associates, Fort Wayne, Indiana
  - Chapter Seven: St. Clair Specialty Physicians, P.C., Detroit, Michigan
  - Chapter Eight: Winthrop University Hospital, Division of Nephrology and Hypertension, Long Island, New York
- Chapter Nine discusses our policy and clinical recommendations for advancing the treatment of CKD.

CHAPTER TWO

Overview of Findings

In this chapter, we provide an overview of key themes and other findings from the 2006 telephone interviews and 2007 case studies. As noted in Chapter One, our evaluation of the 2003 CKDI list of 19 barriers to improved patient outcomes in CKD (Table 1.2) helped us identify topics to be covered in the telephone survey and case studies. The list emphasized specific aspects of both the delivery and financing of care for CKD as prominent barriers to advancing care for this vulnerable population, and our evaluation found that most of these barriers were still in place in 2008.

The 2006–2007 telephone interviews and surveys provide descriptive examples of the challenges faced by CKD practices and clinics, as well as efforts to address these challenges and to improve patient outcomes for kidney disease. These findings established the foundation for a set of policy recommendations in Chapter Nine.

Findings from Telephone Interviews

Prior to performing the case studies, we conducted telephone interviews with leadership from 14 CKD practices or clinics, and one with a staff member from RPA.

A review of findings from the interviews identified the following key themes. We provide examples of each theme below.

Most practices favor early intervention. On the value of intervening at early CKD stages (1 and 2) compared with later stages (3 and 4), six clinics and practices favored early intervention, three were ambivalent, and two stated that payoff was greater only in later stages. Comments tended to focus on prevention. One nephrologist said, "The critical message is now a preventive message. Ten or twelve years ago, there was no evidence that good diabetes control slowed the disease, nor that early control of hypertension slowed disease. Now we know that we should monitor blood sugar, [and] the evidence is quite good that if one controls diabetes one can prevent its sequelae diseases. Also, for even moderately high blood pressure, we can slow the disease, and if we can control blood pressure we can prevent the disease."

A number of "problems or challenges" in treating CKD patients were identified, of which limited reimbursement was primary. The main concern described by clinicians was limited reimbursement for CKD care. Other concerns dealt with patients, including the lack of patient awareness of CKD, challenges in identifying CKD patients, the difficulty of creating patient histories from multiple sources, and patient difficulty in obtaining medications and adhering to prescribed treatments; these concerns were deemed more severe for minority patients.

Relations between nephrologists and other medical specialists—PCPs (internists, family practitioners), cardiologists, and endocrinologists—elicited a good deal of comment. One respondent said, "The interface between internal medicine and nephrology involves some philosophical issues of who should do what." These issues vary as a function of whether nephrologists are located within a hospital, in a general group practice, or in a nephrology practice; as context varies, so do relations with other specialists and so do referral relations.

In general, nephrologists felt that patients were being referred for CKD care too late, although respondents also noted a recent trend toward earlier referrals. An increase in the number of eGFR procedures that are being reimbursed has led to a corresponding increase in the number of early referrals. Some referrals resulted from nephrologists' outreach to specialists in other fields, while others resulted from specialists' recognition of the value of early referrals. Although improved early detection has its advantages, the increased sensitivity of eGFR has led to a rising number of "false positive" diagnoses of CKD and an increased number of referrals to an already overburdened nephrology workforce. The tenuous balance in this setting is not trivial and requires close monitoring.

The organization of CKD care is clearly in flux. Some nephrology practices lack any formal approach to CKD care: "We are a typical office practice," one respondent commented. "We provide CKD care in the old-fashioned way." Other practices had a CKD emphasis but lacked a clear organization and spoke of the need for "a new model of care" or for "changing the culture of our practice" to include training of nurses and establishing the appropriate balance between "right patients" and "wrong patients," i.e., those inappropriately identified as CKD patients. Still others had formally established CKD clinics. One consideration mentioned by some interviewees was the possibility of expanding a quasi-renal workforce through the use of certified nurse practitioners, physician assistants, and others who might bridge the gap for CKD care as well as for other common chronic medical conditions.

In short, interviewees tended to favor intervention at CKD stages 1 and 2, though ambivalence and contrary views strongly suggest the need for clarifying clinical research on the effectiveness of this approach. The primary challenge faced by the respondents was reimbursement for CKD care, which remains the case today. The organization of care remains in flux, with relations with other specialists central to establishing referral of CKD patients before they require ESRD care, usually by dialysis. These findings from the telephone interviews provided invaluable guidance for the site visits we conducted, as the case study findings below indicate.

Findings from Case Studies

The case studies allowed us to build on our understanding of the challenges of CKD care and the ways in which CKD clinics and practices are addressing these issues. These case studies are not intended to be representative of CKD practices in general. In fact, only a small set of nephrology practices and clinics currently focus on CKD care. The practices described in this study are at the front end of the movement to provide CKD care before patients progress to ESRD.

In a publication in 2008, we identified the following overarching conclusions from the case studies:[42]

- The conceptual understanding of CKD is recent and relatively limited within nephrology, medicine, and the health care system.
- The need exists for information on variations in the processes, outcomes, and best practices of CKD care.
- Payers have shown an unwillingness to invest in CKD care.
- A lack of coordination in CKD care exists between nephrologists and PCPs.
- There is an absence of public and patient awareness about the risks of CKD, and of the associated cardiovascular risks of CKD.
- A coordinated system of care that reaches all CKD patients does not exist.
- Information technology systems for CKD care are inadequate.
- Large dialysis organizations have an incentive to view CKD as a feeder stream for ESRD care.

A key reason for conducting the case studies was to understand how these issues play out in individual practices and clinics.

Challenges for and Benefits of Chronic Kidney Disease Clinics and Practices

The case studies that appear in Chapters Three through Eight of this report provide a richness of detail about these findings and shed light in particular on the following challenges that CKD clinics face, as well as some of the ways in which clinics are addressing these challenges.

Reimbursement. In the detailed case studies, as in the telephone interviews, the major barrier to clinic operations involved limitations on reimbursement of CKD. All six of the CKD clinics and practices face financial challenges in providing CKD care, especially to support the multidisciplinary staff of nurses and other health professionals needed for a comprehensive practice.

However, federal reimbursement of CKD care is provided for ESRD but not for effective preventive care. Moreover, the availability of revenues from other ESRD sources care is shrinking, further reducing the incentives to nephrologists to provide CKD care. Reimbursement for preventive "upstream care" by a multidisciplinary approach to CKD care—involving nutritionists, exercise physiologists, dieticians, social workers, and midlevel providers—is critical to reduce costly chronic care interventions.*

Patient Referral. Patient referral remains the second major "resource" question, requiring development of effective working relations with other specialists and, importantly, patient education and community awareness. When a "doorstep patient" arrives at an ESRD facility, the need for dialysis is incontrovertible. But asymptomatic individuals without information about CKD may know virtually nothing about their situation until ESRD care is required.

All CKD clinics and practices have confronted the need to reach out to PCPs, cardiologists, and endocrinologists to ensure the predictable referral of patients for CKD care before patients need immediate dialysis. There was concern among nephrologists that PCPs were reluctant to refer for fear of losing patients, but this concern was tempered in academic and integrated CKD clinics by targeted efforts to comanage CKD with PCPs.

---

* We made no effort to analyze currently proposed reimbursement changes for ESRD, as our field research occurred in 2008.

Patient Screening. The ability to screen potential CKD patients varied across clinics but was generally limited by weak referral patterns in nonintegrated health systems and limited public awareness of the need for early-stage care. The use of eGFR and community outreach programs was cited as a factor in increasing early-stage referrals.

Patient Education. The need to educate both patients and PCPs is critical, both to increase patient awareness of CKD and to ensure that physicians know the early indications of CKD. All CKD clinics engaged in some educational efforts. The range of educational efforts included patient education, e.g., through presentations by nurse educators; community education, e.g., through local talks and media public service announcements; and provider education, e.g., through dinners for PCPs and protocols to assist decisionmaking.

Practice Organization. Clinic organization is quite varied and remains in flux. Because CKD clinics are relatively new, there are uncertainties about how best to structure CKD practices in relation to other medical facilities and organizations to ensure continuity of care through all stages of CKD. The structure of practice organizations in our case studies varied greatly among the six CKD clinics studied. Some nephrology divisions of large multispecialty group practices had carved out a CKD clinic within that context (Northwestern, the Mayo Clinic). In other cases, the CKD effort was an extension of a clinical base in ESRD (AIN, Detroit, Ft. Wayne, Winthrop).

Use of Clinical Practice Guidelines. To ensure high-quality CKD care to those who need it, data are needed on variations in the processes, outcomes, and best practices of CKD care. Guidance is increasingly available through continuously updated clinical practice guidelines. All CKD clinics in our study used the clinical practice guidelines as a first-order means to identify patients, organize practices, and build data systems. All of the clinics visited adapted the guidelines for local and patient-specific purposes.

Health Information Technology. The use of health information technology (HIT) can facilitate CKD care. The six CKD clinics varied greatly in the stage of development of their HIT systems. Some have purchased off-the-shelf products, while others have developed their own. One site received financial assistance from a state and federal government effort to encourage the transition to electronic medical records.

CKD Disparities. Unfortunately, racial and ethnic disparities that are prevalent in the ESRD population appear also in the CKD population, but, without reimbursement, established referral patterns, and high levels of patient knowledge, they often go undetected. In our case studies, sites that served predominantly minority and underserved communities had patients presenting at much younger ages and with more advanced disease. In response, they employed targeted community outreach and educational programs, which included partnerships with organizations such as the National Black Nurses Association and the American Heart Association (AHA) to leverage support for community-based programs.

Benefits of CKD Clinics. The case studies also revealed a number of benefits that flow from CKD clinics.

- Several clinic directors noted that one of the most dramatic motivators of the need for early treatment was the recognition that some of the patients coming for dialysis today were the sons and daughters of their patients of 20 years earlier. Earlier attention to treatable risk factors could have interrupted this tragic flow.
- The clinics reported that the calculation of eGFRs was increasingly resulting in earlier referrals: Approximately 40 percent of laboratory tests now include eGFR.

- Preemptive kidney transplantation, i.e., transplantation before a patient was placed on dialysis, was increasingly possible as a result of the CKD clinics.

The value of these case studies, in our judgment, lies in the information they provide about specific identified CKD clinics and practices and the day-to-day challenges these organizations confront in their efforts to deliver CKD care. Practically speaking, we believe these case studies reveal both commonalities and differences in the provision of CKD care. They also highlight major issues that need to be addressed if a rational foundation for CKD care is to be established, and provide lessons and insights for CKD providers in diverse practice settings. We hope these insights will assist other providers in creating cost-effective practices that will benefit all patients.

Conclusion

This discussion of findings from the interviews and case studies provides an overview of some of the key issues faced by CKD clinics today. In the chapters that follow, we present detailed descriptions of each of the six clinics and practices that participated in the case studies.

CHAPTER THREE

The Chronic Kidney Disease Clinic at Northwestern University, Chicago, Illinois

Richard A. Rettig, Ph.D.;* Daniel Batlle, M.D.; James Paparello, M.D.; Cybele Ghossein, M.D.; Roberto B. Vargas, M.D., M.P.H.; and Allen R. Nissenson, M.D.

The Chronic Kidney Disease Clinic at Northwestern University is a Midwestern urban single-facility practice within an academic department of internal medicine located in downtown Chicago. It serves as a local and outlying suburban referral center, which made a conscious shift in 2000 to improve pre-ESRD care after seeing many late referrals. In 2002, the clinic incorporated preemptive transplantation protocols into the practice, and in 2004 it hired a full-time multidisciplinary team to address the range of CKD patient needs. Processes of care combine patient outreach programs, patient and PCP education, and care coordination of referrals. The academic setting has allowed for a lesser emphasis on profitability and has reduced concerns among referring physicians about losing patients to the clinic. The clinic has a patient registry and has noted encouraging trends in patient outcomes, including stabilization of GFR over a two-year period. However, clinic leaders expressed concern that investments in expanded services such as these need to be balanced against research, academic, and fiscal responsibilities.

Practice Overview

The Northwestern University CKD clinic, called the Healthy Living Clinic (HLC), is an integral part of the Division of Nephrology and Hypertension at the Department of Internal Medicine of the Feinberg School of Medicine, Northwestern University. The clinic is located within the academic complex of the medical school and Northwestern Memorial Hospital in downtown Chicago.

The clinic draws patients from among those who obtain medical services from the Northwestern Medical Faculty Foundation and Northwestern Memorial Hospital. The referral base for this clinic is downtown Chicago and nearby suburbs to the north and south of Chicago.

---

*   This case study is based on site visit interviews conducted on May 2, 2007, supplemented by later correspondence, and preceded by a telephone survey interview of Dr. Daniel Batlle, on May 9, 2006. The site visit and telephone interview were conducted by Dr. Rettig.

Origins and Development of the Clinic

The Northwestern CKD clinic began in 2000 as a comprehensive renal clinic, one of the first of its kind in the country. The clinic developed over two phases. Before 2002, Northwestern nephrologists saw many late referrals, so the focus of CKD treatment was to provide pre-ESRD care. Clinic services consisted primarily of providing education on renal replacement therapy, nutritional counseling, referral for access placement, and anemia management. As the patient population increased, additional services were added.

In 2002 the clinic began to expand and established a protocol-based system of care for patients. These protocols mirrored the guidelines set forth by KDOQI for the care of CKD patients. By 2004, the staff of the CKD clinic was well established, and staff included a full-time physician assistant (PA), two registered nurses (RNs), a licensed practical nurse (LPN), and a renal dietician.

Ghossein et al. described the establishment of the clinic in a review paper in *Seminars in Nephrology*. The authors emphasized the importance of early referral of patients with CKD to nephrologists:[43]

> The decision to establish the clinic was based on several important facts. Our ESRD population was growing, but the patients were being referred to the nephrology service late in the course of their disease. As a result, the ability to intervene was hindered and patients were often starting dialysis before adequate preparation. This lack of preparation was evidenced not only by their suboptimal state of health, but just as importantly by their lack of understanding about the dialysis process itself. The clinic's goal has been to provide a comprehensive approach to the management of chronic kidney failure to ensure that patients starting on dialysis are physically healthier, emotionally prepared, and educated about the process before initiation.

The goal of the CKD clinic today is to provide comprehensive care for patients with renal disease. For late-stage CKD patients, the clinic treats the complications of kidney disease, such as anemia and bone disease; manages the cardiovascular risk factors of CKD patients; and prepares patients for either dialysis or kidney transplantation. For early-stage CKD patients, the clinic attempts to slow the progression of CKD by aggressive treatment of blood pressure, appropriate utilization of ACE inhibitors and ARBs, and treatment of proteinuria and hyperlipidemia.

The nephrologists at the CKD clinic believe that, although good internists are capable of managing CKD patients, physicians who treat CKD patients frequently can do so more effectively. Nephrologists are well versed at addressing the factors that help slow the progression of CKD. CKD physicians are more familiar with complications such as anemia and bone disease and more experienced at treating these complications.[44] In addition, a nephrologist's experience helps guide patients through the choice of renal replacement therapies. In collaboration with the internist, a nephrologist can also treat cardiovascular risk factors.

In addition to better preparing CKD patients for dialysis, the HLC provides preemptive kidney transplant, which follows a diagnosis that renal replacement therapy is needed but before dialysis is required. In 2003–2004, clinic personnel met with transplant surgeons, social workers, and nurses to devise a protocol for a more efficient and faster preemptive transplantation work-up for CKD patients with potential living donors. In 2007, about 20 percent of the clinic's stage 5 CKD patients received a preemptive transplant.

Table 3.1 compares two groups of patients—HLC stage 5 CKD predialysis patients and doorstep ESRD patients (who arrived at the clinic with late-stage ESRD). The former choose one of three treatment modalities—hemodialysis, peritoneal dialysis, or preemptive transplantation—once they reach the point where renal replacement therapy is needed. The latter have not been seen previously in the HLC but arrive from a hospital where they have been admitted in such an advanced stage of CKD that they need immediate dialysis. HLC predialysis patients have roughly comparable rates of diabetes and coronary artery disease compared with doorstep patients, but HLC patients include proportionately fewer African-Americans, suggesting that they are seen earlier by a nephrologist or are referred earlier to the clinic by a PCP.[45]

Northwestern physicians describe the CKD clinic as based on a "paradigm shift" in nephrology thinking, one not reflected in their training. The data regarding outcomes from a two-year follow-up of a cohort of CKD patients suggest the need for rethinking the accepted concept that progression of advanced CKD to ESRD is usually inexorable and relatively rapid.[46, 47] The data show that stabilization of GFR over a two-year period can be achieved in many patients with advanced CKD who are treated with erythropoietin in a CKD clinic.[48] More recent results based on a four-year follow-up of a larger cohort show a very low mortality rate for this population with advanced CKD in stages 4 and 5.[49]

Table 3.1
Healthy Living Clinic Chronic Kidney Disease Patients Compared with Doorstep End-Stage Renal Disease Patients

	HLC Patients: Stage 5 CKD			Doorstep ESRD Patients
	Hemodialysis	Peritoneal Dialysis	Preemptive Transplant	Hemodialysis
Average age	59	55	50	56
% African-American	32	0	21	58
% diabetic	62	30	29	52
% with coronary artery disease	38	20	21	33
Months (average) in HLC before ESRD	22	19	18	N/A
CR at RRT (mg/dL)	7.3	9.3	6.3	8.2

NOTES: HLC patients were followed in the clinic for over three months. On reaching ESRD, these patients chose one of three treatment modalities—hemodialysis, peritoneal dialysis, or a preemptive transplant. Non-HLC patients were those ESRD patients who came to the hospital and required hemodialysis. CR = creatine; RRT = renal replacement therapy.

The Northwestern Chronic Kidney Disease Practice

The Patient Population

In 2000, the clinic began to follow a cohort of about 100 patients; at this time, anemia management with erythropoietin stimulating agents (ESAs) was necessary. These patients have been followed prospectively since then. The clinic estimates that over 500 patients have been followed since 2004. The primary diagnosis of cause of CKD is, first, diabetes, then hypertension, followed by a number of glomerular diseases.

The ethnicity data are approximate, but about 55 percent of patients at the clinic are Caucasian and about 45 percent are African-American or Hispanic. About 50 percent of HLC patients come from an impoverished, geographically isolated, minority or non–English-speaking population. During the two-year follow-up of the initial cohort, outcomes were worse among African-Americans: GFR declined more rapidly, progression to ESRD occurred more quickly, dialysis was required earlier, and mortality was higher. Interestingly, at the four-year follow-up, the ethnic differences in mortality were no longer apparent.[50]

Despite the progress, many Northwestern CKD patients, particularly African-American and non–English-speaking populations, are still referred too late. Some progress is being made in this regard, however, with the use of eGFR (the laboratories most commonly used have been calculating eGFR for a year or two). Since the introduction of eGFR, there has been an improvement in the referral pattern, with more patients referred earlier in the course of their disease. The reporting of eGFR along with serum creatinine has helped internists recognize renal disease earlier, and, as a result, they refer earlier.[51]

Outreach, Education, and Referrals

Since the CKD clinic is part of the Northwestern Medical Faculty Foundation, the physician arm of the Feinberg School of Medicine, and is located within the Northwestern Memorial Hospital building, the principal source of patient referrals is Northwestern PCPs within this academic center, as well as voluntary faculty practices associated with Northwestern. Some referrals come from internists in the greater Chicago area.

Within the city of Chicago, Northwestern CKD clinic personnel attend local conferences. They also discuss CKD issues with physicians who refer patients to the hospital. The clinic receives many second-opinion requests from its referral sources. In general, the CKD clinic engages in limited community outreach, although it may increase future efforts in this direction. At present, it does little promotion through local newspapers or television.

As part of a large faculty practice, clinic physicians do not face the same economic concerns often seen in the private sector.[52] Clinicians in faculty practices often receive additional salary support from teaching and research activities. In addition, the nephrologists are not considered to be "stealing" patients from internists and certainly not to be taking money from them. The internists know that the nephrologists are not in private practice and that there are no hidden agendas behind encouraging early referral. In fact, the nephrology practice loses money by caring for CKD patients. The care model requires collaboration with internists, with the nephrologist providing care for kidney disease and the internist providing nonrenal care.

CKD care in a multidisciplinary clinic of this type needs to be promoted within the PCP community. In the view of Northwestern nephrologists, PCPs should recognize that the best quality of care for CKD can be provided by specialists in an integrated system and with support for all needs. The clinic provides services that the individual physician cannot provide alone: Specialized nurses provide anemia management; a renal nutritionist provides diet counseling for kidney disease patients; and specialized PAs provide support while billing independently of the doctors.[53]

This care model, when coupled with better care in general for CKD patients throughout the country, may account for the recent decrease in the number of incident patients entering dialysis programs, as reported by the latest USRDS report. This decrease provides "grounds for optimism," according to the Northwestern group, who believe that kidney disease can be stabilized even in its advanced stages and that this is a message of optimism that should be transmitted to patients and referring physicians.[54]

Clinic Organization

The CKD clinic is housed in a new building within the Northwestern campus in downtown Chicago. The outpatient dialysis unit is also located within the hospital building. All needed renal medical services—CKD, kidney transplantation, and dialysis—are available within this academic complex.

In a 2002 issue of *Seminars in Nephrology*, Ghossein et al. described the Northwestern clinic organization as follows:

> The pre-ESRD team was established with a staff of nephrologists, a physician assistant, nurses, a nutritionist, and access to renal social workers. Each member of the team focuses on different aspects of the comprehensive care with the main objectives being (1) treating the complications of CKD including anemia and renal osteodystrophy; (2) providing nutritional support; (3) identifying and managing comorbidities; (4) preparing for transplantation; and (5) preparing for dialysis.[55]

An electronic medical record was launched in 2004 and has been utilized to help track the established CKD patients.

The clinic originally had one RN, one PA, and seven nephrologists from the Division of Nephrology and Hypertension. Currently it has two nurses, an LPN, a dietitian, and one and one-half PAs. Over the last several years, seven nephrologists have had their patients managed in the CKD clinic under their supervision. The primary reasons for referral into the clinic are CKD education, management of CKD complications, and overall renal care. Once patients have been referred into the clinic, the PA sees them on a regular basis.

Clinic Procedures

Patients are staged in terms of eGFR using the formula developed by the Modification of Diet in Renal Disease (MDRD) clinical trial. The Northwestern Hospital laboratory calculates eGFR routinely, as do other laboratories used by the clinic.

Once a physician diagnoses kidney disease, the patient is sent to a nephrologist for initial evaluation. Once the nephrologist has established the diagnosis of CKD, he or she refers the patient to the PA for initial CKD education and treatment. Treatment differs according to CKD stage:

- Stage 2 patients (eGFR 60–89) and stage 3a patients (eGFR 45–60) are usually seen annually once their proteinuria and blood pressure are under control.

- Stage 3b patients (eGFR 30–44) are seen as often as needed until their blood pressure and proteinuria are at goal. Then they are seen every six months or as deemed necessary by the physician or PA.
- Stage 4 patients (eGFR 15–29) are seen every three months for a follow-up appointment with the PA. The nurses will often see these patients weekly or every other week if they are being treated for anemia. They represent a smaller percentage of CKD patients but a greater percentage of visits. For example, anemia management will be required to address issues and to ask about individual patient concerns.

CKD patients receive nutritional counseling from a renal dietitian at several times on follow-up visits to the clinic—"initially at a GFR of 30–50 mL/min. and then again at a GFR of 20–25 mL/min."[56] The information conveyed is both theoretical and practical, concerning the risk of malnutrition and review of patient's dietary intake and appetite.

For new patients, the wait time for a clinic appointment is less than two weeks.

Practice Guidelines

Northwestern nephrologists utilize the 2002 NKF clinical practice guidelines, which they consider crucial to their success in managing CKD patients. Areas of focus include treatment of anemia, renal osteodystrophy, and appropriate referral for transplantation. The guidelines are used extensively to facilitate the work of the RNs and the PAs as well. There is variability as to when the internist refers to the CKD clinic, but once in the clinic, there is a consistency of care.[57]

Ghossein added,

> We are always reevaluating the protocols. For example, hemoglobin (Hgb) is under regular review. We are conservative, in the 11–12 range for the last year or so. We modified the calcium phosphorous guidelines; they were too stringent. On calcium phosphorous/PTH we had to adjust the guidelines. It was a question of priorities. There is so much to deal with, so much going on in the patients' lives: e.g., high blood pressure, diabetes care, anemia for low hemoglobin, vascular access, early listing for preemptive transplantation.[58]

Treatment Outcomes

The Northwestern CKD clinic has reported on a prospective study of a cohort of 82 patients with advanced CKD in stages 4 and 5.[59] These patients were entered into a database on a consecutive, unselected basis. The primary intervention was protocol-based erythropoietin therapy, which initiated the two-year follow-up period. Primary outcomes measured were the initiation of renal replacement therapy by dialysis or kidney transplantation, and death. For patients who did not attain these outcomes, the main study endpoint was the level of GFR estimated using the MDRD formula.

The ethnicity of the patients in this initial cohort was as follows: African-American, 40 percent; Caucasian, 51 percent; and other, 9 percent. The mean age was 64.8 years, with a range of 26–102 years. Forty-three percent were male. Diabetes was present in 40 percent of patients and hypertension in 80 percent. Of the 47 patients who did not reach a primary outcome at the end of two years, their eGFR "remained essentially unchanged."[60] Thirty-eight of these individuals were stage 4 patients, and nine were stage 5.

External Relations

Reimbursement

A fundamental issue for all CKD clinics is to determine how CKD care is and should be financed. Stages 3 and 4 of CKD are recognized as diagnostic entities. However, billing is tied to the procedure, not to the recognized diagnosis.

The Northwestern clinic faces reimbursement challenges similar to those seen in private practice clinics. Billing can occur only for the physician's fee and the PA's fee. There is no mechanism to bill for nurses and the countless phone calls they receive throughout the day. The nursing staff is financed at the clinic's expense, resulting in a financial loss to the nephrology division.

The clinic's relations with health insurers are typical of those of any outpatient practice. Despite careful billing, the clinic, which has substantial overhead, recovers only a very small portion of the amount billed. The net result is a financial loss, but the work continues because of the importance of providing good medical care to those who need it.

Future Challenges

The major challenge that the Northwestern University CKD clinic faces is to establish sufficient reimbursement mechanisms to ensure that providing CKD care is economically feasible.

A second challenge is to expand the clinic. Although there are economic reasons arguing against expansion, the clinic has expansion plans. An expanded clinic would support the provision of good nephrology care, facilitate the physicians' work, and create a research opportunity for clinical faculty and visibility for the institution.

CHAPTER FOUR

Associates in Nephrology, Chicago, Illinois

Richard A. Rettig, Ph.D.; Paul W. Crawford, M.D.; Roberto B. Vargas, M.D., M.P.H.; and
Allen R. Nissenson, M.D.*

Associates in Nephrology (AIN) is a Midwestern urban single-specialty community practice with multiple sites serving a predominantly African-American patient population on the southwest side of Chicago. The practice receives referrals mainly from local private practices and HMOs. At its inception, the group initially focused on ESRD care, but it was soon compelled to develop a CKD practice, as the practice observed that there were seldom any treatment options left for many of the patients being referred. The practice rapidly developed a high demand for services and has evolved into a multidisciplinary care team including a nurse practitioner (NP), dietician, and social worker. However, the added costs to provide these services are not covered by current reimbursement. The practice aims to balance prevention and treatment by emphasizing outreach, education, and promotion of lifestyle changes to patients at all stages. The practice clinician champion of this effort has a visible presence in the community through church-based programs, local media, and collaborations with nonprofit public health groups. There is also a concerted outreach effort to primary care practices that aims to encourage referrals at earlier stages. The practice maintains a disease registry and collects observational data on delayed progression and, in some cases, reversal of CKD. However, staff expressed the need to expand the electronic billing records to incorporate clinical data and to develop financial support to pay for multidisciplinary team care for early-stage patients.

Practice Overview

The AIN practice is a single-specialty group nephrology practice located in the Chicago metropolitan area. The practice includes 27 board-certified nephrologists who follow patients at 34 hemodialysis clinics, 21 Fresenius Medical Care (FMC) clinics, and 11 nursing homes. In 2007, AIN physicians saw 1,650 ESRD patients and more than 3,000 CKD patients. In addition, the practice cares for 195 patients with transplants, 32 on continuous cycler peritoneal dialysis (CCPD), 29 on continuous ambulatory peritoneal dialysis (CAPD), and two on home dialysis.

The AIN practice includes two CKD clinics. The first is located in the Evergreen Park neighborhood on the southwest side of Chicago, in the same building that houses the FMC Evergreen Park Dialysis Unit. The Evergreen Park CKD practice includes seven nephrologists

---

* This case study is based on an extended site visit interview conducted by Dr. Rettig on May 1, 2007, and supplemented by later correspondence; the site visit was preceded by a telephone survey interview conducted by Dr. Rettig with Dr. Paul W. Crawford on April 10, 2006.

and handles the majority of CKD patient referrals to the group. A second prevention clinic is located in the northern suburb of Park Ridge near Lutheran General Hospital and is staffed by three nephrologists. Paul W. Crawford, M.D., a physician partner of AIN, is also the medical director of the Evergreen Park Dialysis Unit of FMC and of several other dialysis units.

The Evergreen Park AIN urban practice draws the majority of its patients from the area; many come from the Advocate Health Care system. Other patient referral sources include PCPs at local hospitals, local community PCPs, and HMOs. AIN patients are primarily African-American, but the ethnic distribution varies by location. Although the practice is located at some distance from a major Hispanic population, the group recently hired a Spanish-speaking physician to better serve Hispanic patients.

Origins and Development of the Clinic

In 1979, Dr. Paul Crawford, an African-American nephrologist trained in Chicago, joined AIN, which at that time owned four dialysis units and a nephrology practice. He chose to practice in the community where he had been raised. At the time, dialysis units were successfully established in communities served by a number of small south side hospitals, including South Chicago Community, South Shore, Hyde Park, Roseland Community, and Provident hospitals. As the practice grew, it focused chiefly on ESRD patient care, and little attention was initially paid to prevention of CKD or care for predialysis CKD patients. The AIN dialysis practice was a part of Neomedica, a small dialysis chain that owned 20 dialysis units, until 1998. In that year, the dialysis clinic part of Neomedica, which had become attractive to the large corporate dialysis chains, was sold to FMC.

The AIN CKD practice began after members of the practice examined the current paradigm of care and considered what additional services were needed in the community. Traditionally, nephrologists saw kidney disease as a progressive disease that inevitably led to ESRD and dialysis or transplantation. At the time of AIN's inception, no one in nephrology was talking about prevention. PCPs functioning in the fee-for-service environment would wait until creatinine was elevated to 4.0 mg/dL or greater before referring a patient to a nephrologist. The advent of managed care added to this problem, as PCPs became even more reluctant to refer patients early to a nephrologist, fearing loss of control and capitated income. By the time referrals were made, there were seldom any treatment options except dialysis or transplant. Although the harmful effects of late referral had been well documented in the literature for ten years, there were still no data available to support the value of early intervention.[61]

AIN decided to open a CKD clinic and hired a secretary-receptionist to manage the administrative side of the practice. There were no nurses initially, and the nephrologists did all patient intake. As the practice grew, an NP was hired to help with patient intake and other tasks, including patient education. The practice became more efficient and received more referrals, subsequently expanding its community outreach activities.

Although initially the clinic focused on slowing the progression of CKD, or smoothing the transition to ESRD, the emphasis later shifted to preventing premature death from cardiovascular disease in patients with CKD as well as stabilizing and reversing progression. AIN physicians believe that the majority of CKD cases are preventable, i.e., that high blood pressure and diabetes do not have to lead to dialysis.

Halting the inheritance of kidney disease within families is one of the goals of AIN. Dr. Crawford tells a dramatic human story about what prompted the initiation of the CKD practice:

> In the dialysis unit, I am now treating *the children* of my first dialysis patients. I have mother-daughter and father-son dialysis patients. This is often due to uncontrolled but preventable hypertension and diabetes. It is a slap in the face to see these children. This should not happen. Something is wrong with this picture.

As the CKD prevention practice grew, AIN began differentiating the diagnosis and treatment of CKD patients from its ESRD dialysis activity. Initially, it held a renal clinic one-half day per week, but as demand and numbers of referrals increased, clinic days were added until four and one-half days per week were needed to see referrals in a timely fashion.

The Associates in Nephrology Chronic Kidney Disease Practice

CKD practices are in an early stage of development. The AIN CKD practice is engaged simultaneously in developing clinical routines and protocols, creating internal organizational processes, and establishing external relations with those who provide patient referrals and financing of operations. The need to depend on other organizations for referrals makes AIN different from other clinical practices that have a predictable inflow of patients and that treat a range of well-understood diseases.

The Patient Population

The total number of AIN CKD patients, by initial stage of diagnosis, is shown in Table 4.1 for the period from October 2005 to February 2006. Although the billing data do not permit a determination of the primary diagnosis of the cause of CKD from associated comorbid conditions, these data show that 99 percent of patients seen have hypertension, and 97 percent have diabetes. Ethnicity data are not consistently designated on billing information, but it is estimated that minority patients, mostly African-Americans, account for 90 percent of the AIN practice at the Evergreen Park location.

The insurance status of the CKD patients is shown in Table 4.2.

Table 4.1
Number of Chronic Kidney Disease Patients at the Associates in Nephrology Clinic, by Stage of Disease, October 2005–February 2006

CKD Stage	Number of Patients
Stage 1	119
Stage 2	330
Stage 3	1,724
Stage 4	1,518
Stage 5	218

Table 4.2
Insurance Status of Chronic Kidney Disease Patients at the Associates in Nephrology Clinic, October 2005–February 2006

Type of Insurance	Percentage
Medicare	31
Medicaid	7
HMOs	50
PPOs	3
Commercial	8
Self-pay	1

In AIN's experience, a much higher prevalence and more advanced stage of CKD are seen among minorities, especially younger minorities. In this population, young black males have been less willing to deal with asymptomatic, previously undiagnosed hypertension, diabetes, hyperlipidemia, obesity, and the harm caused by smoking. AIN physicians attribute this unwillingness to the "I feel good syndrome," i.e., "if I feel good, how can there be anything wrong with me?" The failure of patients to accept treatment of these comorbidities often results in CKD.

Outreach, Education, and Referrals

Central to any community-based CKD clinic is a steady flow of patients. Consequently, outreach and educational activities designed to promote lifestyle changes and prevention measures and, peripherally, to generate patient referrals are as integral to a CKD clinic as are the clinical procedures used to treat patients.

The AIN CKD practice is built on extensive community outreach and educational efforts, which focus on prevention of kidney disease, heart disease, diabetes, and other conditions. Crawford has participated in volunteer work through community organizations, especially African-American churches. Minority education efforts have been conducted in conjunction with the American Kidney Fund (AKF) in Chicago, Washington, D.C., and Atlanta.

Dr. Crawford was instrumental in founding the Church Based Hypertension Program of the Chicago chapter of the AHA, which initially screened for hypertension and later for urine, creatinine, and metabolic disorders. This program became the basis for the AHA's national Search Your Heart outreach program and has encouraged more comprehensive health ministries. Dr. Crawford has also worked with the National Black Nurses Association, put on health fairs, and participated in the Kidney Mobile Van for Illinois program, sponsored by the NKF of Illinois. Frequent radio and TV spots and interviews increase the reach of the practice and provide the community with education regarding CKD.

Part of outreach focuses on other medical specialties. PCPs are the primary source of referrals to the CKD clinic. The CKD clinic has strengthened relations with those who make referrals, focusing on PCPs who continue to refer patients late, in stage 4 or 5. Significant barriers to early referral persist, caused in part by the nephrology community itself. PCPs report that they have sent patients to nephrologists with early CKD as indicated by NKF's KDOQI guidelines, only to have the nephrologist question why the patient was sent. "The key is to get

PCPs and patients to understand CKD care as preventive nephrology, not pre-ESRD nephrology," Dr. Crawford said.

In general, relationships with medical subspecialists and PCPs are good. Reciprocal referrals may be an important component of relationships with other specialists, particularly with cardiologists. Endocrinologists, on the other hand, tend to be less aggressive with diabetes management in CKD patients, and nephrologists are increasingly managing this important comorbidity.

AIN physicians believe that many CKD patients are still referred too late to the CKD clinic, although early-stage referrals seem to be increasing. The timing of referral appears to be generational: Younger or more recently trained M.D.'s tend to refer early, while some older doctors have not changed or updated their practice patterns, or may not have the database or staff to help them manage their patients as effectively.

In a poster presentation at the NKF clinical meeting in the spring of 2006, AIN presented data showing the change over time in the source of referrals of patients for treatment of ESRD.[62] In 1995, 88 percent of referrals for ESRD treatment came from hospitals, and only 12 percent came from the CKD clinic. That proportion held relatively constant through 2000. It then fell steadily from 2001 through 2005. In 2005, fewer than half of ESRD referrals came from hospitals (41 percent), and 59 percent came from the CKD clinic. This shift reflects an increase in patients who receive earlier preparation for dialysis treatment and a decrease in those presenting from a hospital emergency room. An increase in early referrals has increased the number of preemptive transplants and the ease of starting patients on home dialysis modalities. When a late referral results in emergency hemodialysis, it is much more difficult to convert a patient to another dialysis mode.

Regarding the relative importance of early-stage (stage 1 or 2) interventions versus late-stage (stage 3 or 4) CKD interventions for slowing progression to ESRD, AIN is not entirely in agreement with the NKF guidelines. Dr. Crawford said:

> Some interpret the guidelines as suggesting that referral to the nephrologist is not needed until the GFR is <60 mL/min; others interpret them as requiring referral at <30 mL/min. Earlier referral provides greater opportunity to slow progression or even to improve GFR. I think it's a missed opportunity to stabilize and/or improve GFR. There is a significant population that has some reversible component of kidney disease. A nephrologist is best prepared to address the issues of preventive nephrology. In the majority of patients in stages 1–4, stabilization of kidney function is possible.

Clinic Organization

The Evergreen Park CKD clinic includes an administrative assistant, a receptionist, and two medical assistants. There are now seven nephrologists associated with the clinic, an increase from three nephrologists just two years earlier. FMC shares the expense of the NP. FMC also uses the services of a dietitian in CKD classes to educate patients about nutrition.

The clinic has three examination rooms and an 8–10 patient capacity waiting room. At the time of the interview, a major office expansion was underway. The expansion increased the clinic's size from 900 square feet to 2,500 square feet, with six exam rooms and a waiting room capacity of 25. The expansion was based on a projected doubling of the number of patients.

Health Information Technology System

The clinic has a limited electronic record system for billing purposes but not for tracking patients. There is no clinical data system, although one is planned.

Clinic Procedures

Staging of CKD is based on the MDRD equation for estimating GFR. Some laboratories are starting to report eGFR but are not required to do so by Illinois law. There are efforts to change this, and some hospitals calculate eGFRs, but AIN generally does its own calculations. The sources of resistance to calculating eGFR include pathologists who complain about not having the right equipment and PCPs who say that explaining GFR to patients is difficult.

The patient wait time for an initial appointment is long but is continually being improved. Typically, patients wait 2–3 months for an appointment, although urgent cases are seen quickly. The waiting time is partly driven by a philosophy at AIN to reject the common practice among nephrologists of backing away from complete care for the kidney disease patient in order to do consults instead, thus not establishing a continued patient-physician relationship. In contrast, AIN nephrologists do comprehensive evaluations and detailed work-ups of patients. Based on these evaluations, patients and PCPs are advised on aspects of care related to comorbid conditions as well as the CKD.

AIN has education programs on nutrition for all patients; for early-stage patients (stages 1, 2, and 3), there are monthly classes on nutrition and diet. A significant percentage of CKD patients who are followed for several years before reaching CKD stage 5 receive preemptive transplants. Monthly classes on renal replacement therapy are held for stage 4 patients and for diabetic patients. Late stage 4 or stage 5 patients, usually men, often come in because their spouses insist that they see a doctor. Many of these men put up a lot of resistance and reflect a good deal of denial. A major educational effort is needed for these patients, and some require confrontation. Patients often have cardiovascular problems that are more ominous than kidney disease problems. With late referrals, everything is "shock therapy."

Practice Guidelines

AIN uses the NKF CKD and RPA CKD toolkits to assist in CKD care. However, more important are the people that implement the toolkits. The tools cannot be used appropriately without dedicated nephrologists and staff. The use of multidisciplinary teams is a key component of the AIN CKD practice.

Treatment Outcomes

The AIN practice believes it is possible to slow progression or stabilize CKD in many of their patients and to reverse it in some patients. In 2003, based on data from 2001–2002, AIN looked at several hundred CKD patients and found either a slowing of kidney disease or a stabilizing of the disease for the majority of patients. These data also showed that regression of CKD was achieved in some patients. For patients followed one year or more, 53 percent were stabilized, 29 percent got worse, and 18 percent improved. AIN believes that the later a patient is referred, the less potential to slow the disease's progression. AIN physicians believe that they could slow or halt progression in half of CKD patients if referred early.

Although these data have not yet been published, a more recent analysis of 431 AIN patients followed for one year or more was conducted in 2005–2006, based on billing data only from one unit, and the results were presented at the 2007 NKF Spring Clinical Meeting.

The sample included both diabetic and nondiabetic patients, 30 percent of whom got worse (progressed to an additional stage), 53 percent of whom were unchanged (stabilized), and 17 percent of whom improved (reverted one CKD stage).[63] In a retrospective analysis of patients cared for by both PCPs and nephrologists, those patients cared for in nephrology-led CKD clinics maintained hemoglobin levels within the KDOQI guidelines range of 11–12 mg/dL better than those cared for by PCPs, improved other biochemical outcomes, and slowed progression of kidney disease.[64]

External Relations

Reimbursement

The key issue for AIN, as for all CKD clinics, is reimbursement. AIN leaders believe that nephrologists must be compensated for the prevention of CKD. Most income is generated from acute care dialysis in the hospital and chronic dialysis in the dialysis clinic, but, from a public health perspective, CKD care should be supported. AIN loses money on its CKD practice and has difficulty meeting the expenses of the NP, dietitian, social worker, and others. Many nephrologists are adamant that CKD clinics should not bear the extra expense of an NP. The collaboration with FMC CKD Services has been more helpful for AIN in improving patient care and achieving excellent outcomes in managing hypertension, anemia, and diabetes and improving GFR than the financial balance sheet will justify. These results would not have been achievable without the help of a multidisciplinary team including NPs, dietitians, and social workers. The real test of the financial viability of the CKD clinic will come from the expansion described earlier. It remains to be seen whether the financial reward of the expansion will outweigh the financial risk.

Reimbursement is still limited to procedures, not prevention. For example, an interventional nephrology unit that provides services for late-stage patients—vein mapping, catheter insertion, maintaining and preserving fistulas, and procedures for vascular access—can earn more in half a day than the AIN clinic can in a week of CKD care.

The relevant private health insurers include Blue Cross Blue Shield of Illinois, Humana, Cigna, Aetna, Unicare, and UnitedHealthcare. Policies of these payers are reasonable regarding physician services, but there are serious issues with restrictive formularies. Illinois Medicaid is a reasonable payer as well, although there are long delays between billing and actual payment.

AIN has corporate relations exclusively with FMC, one of the two largest dialysis treatment corporations in the country. AIN provides the medical directors for 18–20 FMC units. FMC had not been doing CKD care but wanted to get into the business. FMC and AIN share a nurse practitioner, with each group paying for the portion of time and expertise used.

Future Challenges

AIN faces many challenges, the most important of which is inadequate reimbursement. There is also a need for a full-time nurse practitioner. The second challenge is late referrals, which reflect physicians' and patients' lack of understanding of kidney disease. A third challenge involves patients who are afraid of or confused about kidney disease for cultural or psychosocial reasons, or patients who are referred but who never come for evaluation. As explained by

Dr. Crawford, "Almost all African-Americans have a past or current family member or friend on dialysis, and they have minimal knowledge of and fear of dialysis. The word on the street is 'Stay away from the kidney doctor; he will put you on dialysis.' We need to change the general public perception of kidney disease."

An additional challenge identified by Dr. Crawford concerns inadequate systems for collecting and analyzing data on a practice level. Data are needed to publicly document the practice's experience for internal use to improve the outcomes and efficiencies of care.

CHAPTER FIVE

Mayo Clinic Nephrology, Jacksonville, Florida

Richard A. Rettig, Ph.D.; William E. Haley, M.D.; Peter M. Fitzpatrick, M.D.;*
Jamie P. Dwyer, M.D.; Roberto B. Vargas, M.D., M.P.H.; and Allen R. Nissenson, M.D.

The Mayo Clinic has locations in Minnesota, Arizona, and Florida. This case is based on the Mayo Clinic in Jacksonville, Florida, which serves a broad region of the southeastern United States and is a large referral center. Within the clinic, the nephrology division receives referrals from a broad geographic region and a neighboring state, with 25 percent of kidney patients referred from outside of the Mayo system. Roughly 40 percent of patients are one- to two-time visit consultations. Fewer than 15 percent of patients are from minority groups. The Mayo Clinic's decision to develop a CKD clinic within the nephrology division was concurrent with the 2002 publication of CKD guidelines. The design was driven by financial viability, with a strong emphasis on highlighting noncompetitive, tertiary, and quaternary care to referring PCPs. Within the Mayo system, CKD education is emphasized for PCPs, and the practice model protocols focus primarily on stage 4–5 patients and use a centralized scheduling process. An electronic medical record with integrated clinical guidelines provides decision support. Future challenges include the need for greater screening, improved care by non-nephrologists, and a balance between increased demand for nephrologists' services and limited financial support for care for a growing CKD population.

Practice Overview

The Mayo Clinic in Jacksonville, Florida, a large multispecialty practice, serves a geographically diverse population through an outpatient campus facility located on the southeastern side of Jacksonville. Until April 2008, it also provided services at St. Luke's Hospital several miles to the west; however, Mayo's services were no longer needed after an on-campus hospital opened.

The Mayo Clinic in Jacksonville, Florida, like its Rochester, Minnesota, parent organization, is a major referral treatment center. The patient population it serves comes from many sources: Approximately 50 percent of patients come from northeast Florida, 20 percent from the rest of Florida and Georgia, 10 percent from the rest of the southeastern United States and eastern seaboard, a small percentage from the rest of the United States, and about 10 percent from other countries. The CKD clinic draws patients from the same geographically diverse population base.

* This case study is based on site visit interviews conducted by Dr. Rettig on May 24, 2007, and December 27, 2007, supplemented by email communications; the visits were preceded by an April 6, 2006, telephone interview of Dr. Haley by Dr. Rettig.

The CKD clinic is managed by three nephrologists: William E. Haley, M.D., chair of the Division of Nephrology and Hypertension; Peter M. Fitzpatrick, M.D, director of dialysis services and the chief architect of the CKD clinic; and Jamie P. Dwyer, M.D. Two nephrology NPs participate as members of this collaborative, multidisciplinary CKD team, which also includes a secretary, a dietician, a pharmacist, a vascular surgeon, a nephrology social worker, and the patient's PCP.

Origins and Development of the Clinic

The Mayo CKD clinic emerged in the early 2000s as the result of two developments. The first was the establishment of a collaborative nephrology practice using NPs as physician extenders to increase productivity while assuring quality care. The teamwork model among physicians and nurses, NPs, and PAs enables the CKD clinic to work efficiently. The benefits of such teamwork included improved patient care, increased patient and staff satisfaction, and economic viability.

The second development involved the establishment of an explicit approach to CKD care. Before the 2002 KDOQI and RPA CKD guidelines were published, the practice focused on ESRD care. CKD patients not needing dialysis were seen, but little focus was placed on these latter patients because of time and resource constraints. To address the growing need to see CKD patients, a special clinic was developed that focused on a common set of needs—hypertension control, nutrition, anemia management, and other predialysis needs. A streamlined clinic, comanaged with NPs and structured for efficiency, was established to allow the clinic to see more patients.

An immediate challenge was the need to show financial viability. A comprehensive financial evaluation pushed the clinic toward the model managed by nephrologists and NPs. (In Florida, it is possible for an NP to bill independently for services; PAs, however, are unable to do so.) But a financially viable practice required a flow of patients and the efficient use of resources to ensure that the clinic did not become a financial drain. The group pilot-tested the clinic concept for several years to establish its financial soundness.

When the 2002 KDOQI and RPA CKD guidelines were published, they were adopted by the clinic and used in the planning efforts and in constructing a template for optimal care. The guidelines identified the essential ingredients to the CKD system, framed the system, and helped drive the organization of the CKD clinic. The CKD guidelines helped provide a template for a standardized CKD clinic visit within a system designed to ensure that multiple and complex issues were addressed in a timely fashion and that the goals of care were accomplished.

The Mayo Clinic Chronic Kidney Disease Practice

The Chronic Kidney Disease Clinic Patient Population

The total number of CKD clinic patients for 2002–2007 is shown in Figure 5.1. The age of patients ranged from 22 to 95 years; the mean age of patients was 70, +/–15 years; 38 percent were female; and 13 percent were African-American. Of the 275 patients in 2007, 139 had GFR greater than 30 on enrollment and 136 had GFR below 30. As of the end of 2007, 96 percent survived, 3 percent were lost to follow-up, and 6 percent had progressed to ESRD.

Figure 5.1
Mayo Clinic, Jacksonville, Chronic Kidney Disease Clinic Population

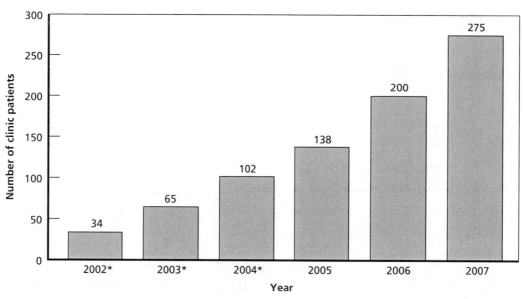

*Pilot-testing phase: 2002–2004.

RAND *TR826-5.1*

The most common cause of CKD among the Mayo population is diabetic kidney disease associated with high blood pressure. Data as of the end of 2007 showed that 39 percent of patients had diabetic CKD and 61 percent had nondiabetic CKD, reflecting the patient referral base. Less common causes of CKD are hypertension alone, other vascular diseases, and other forms of glomerulonephritis. Hypertension is present in most patients with CKD. However, the Mayo patient population may be somewhat skewed because it is a referral center.

The CKD clinic approach focuses much less on the specific cause of CKD than on the CKD stage, comorbidities, and complications. For the 275 patients, comorbidities were as follows: hypertension, 93 percent; diabetes mellitus, 39 percent; hyperlipidemia, 69 percent; and coronary artery disease, 25 percent (see Figure 5.2).

The Mayo patient population is not heavily weighted toward minority groups, which represent approximately 15 percent of all patients. The major difference between minority and nonminority patients lies in the greater incidence of hypertension as a primary cause of CKD. In the nonminority patients, CKD is often part of a set of comorbidities; there is a high prevalence of diabetes, with hypertension secondary. Minority patients are often younger in age, have more advanced CKD, and have a more rapid rate of CKD progression.

Three-quarters of the CKD clinic patients have Medicare as their insurer. For the others, commercial-contract patients account for 15 percent; commercial noncontract patients for 6 percent; and 6 percent have various other forms of insurance (Mayo employees, Medicaid, self-pay, and other government insurance).

The Mayo Clinic CKD practice is primarily designed to focus on stages 4 and 5. This emphasis is based on the fact that by stage 4, symptoms and complications are manifesting, progression is often accelerating, and active management appears to influence outcomes.[65, 66] Given scarce resources, a reasonable point at which regular visits with a nephrologist begin to occur is stage 4 or 5. Providing diagnosis and treatment of the cause of CKD is addressed at the

Figure 5.2
Distribution of Comorbidities Among Patients at the Mayo Clinic

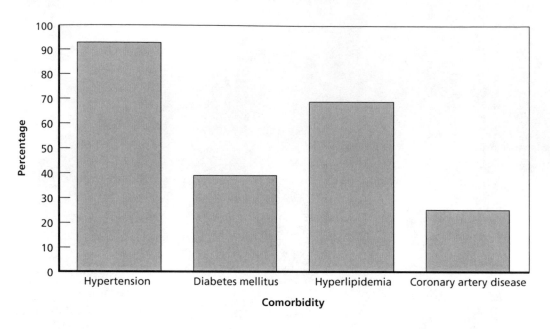

RAND *TR826-5.2*

initial consult, along with recommendations; screening for and treating progression risk factors, comorbidities, and cardiovascular (CV) risk factors; and adjustment of medication doses.

It is well known that late referrals result in poor outcomes for CKD patients, both in progression to ESRD and in first-year mortality on dialysis.[67] This fact has reinforced the Mayo approach that physicians involved in ESRD care also must be involved in CKD care. With the routine calculation of eGFR, an increasing number of early referrals are occurring, especially from family medicine and general internal medicine.

Those patients who fare the worst are those who present at late stages. These include younger minority patients with severe high blood pressure, sometimes in the 200 over 120 range; those suffering from inability to comply with medical management advice and follow-up; and the very elderly (over 75–80 years of age), who are presenting in a very fragile state. The Mayo philosophy is that it is not possible to see a patient too early; nonetheless, patients are often seen too late, e.g., with a history of poor blood pressure control or a history of proteinuria. "For many patients, there is a window of time to treat before progression becomes irreversible. Too often the patients are seen as the window is closing," Dr. Haley noted.

Outreach, Education, and Referrals

Central to any CKD clinic is the establishment of a steady flow of patients. Consequently, outreach and educational activities are as integral to a CKD clinic as are the clinical procedures used to treat patients. However, the nature and philosophy of the Mayo Clinic, including its nephrology division, coupled with its patterns of patient referral, make the CKD clinic distinctive relative to other CKD clinics and practices. Embedded in the Mayo Clinic's organization and philosophy is the goal of partnering with local or distant referring physicians by providing tertiary or quaternary services that are not in competition with these doctors.

Patients are referred to Mayo, as indicated above, from various sources—and to the CKD clinic mostly from within the multispecialty practice itself; from the local Jacksonville area; and from the rest of Florida, the southeastern United States, and the eastern seaboard. The largest source of referrals is internal: the 400 Mayo Clinic physicians in Florida, who include both PCPs and other specialties. Some patients may be local, i.e., from Jacksonville and the immediate surrounding area; some of these, in turn, may be engaged in an ongoing care relationship at Mayo; others may be seen for evaluation and then referred back to their outside physician, either a nephrologist or PCP. Mayo nephrologists also see many nonlocal patients: Some may reside in St. Augustine, 40–45 miles to the south; others may be Florida's "snowbirds," seasonal migrants to Florida from the northern United States, who need to be seen only during three or four months of the year; and still others may be more distant referrals who come only for evaluation. About one-fourth of the CKD clinic patients come from outside referrals, from the northeastern Florida region and beyond.

The number of consultations, therefore, greatly exceeds the number of CKD clinic patients. At the end of 2007, for example, there had been 1,850 consults, of which more than 10 percent were estimated to be pure hypertension evaluation and treatment. More than 1,500 new kidney disease consults were seen in 2007. The CKD clinic population is a select subset of patients seen initially as consults over the past five years, who numbered 275 at the end of 2007.

Comanagement of CKD patients in the Mayo system is a critical issue. Collaborative management with non-nephrologists is emphasized, but a principal concern is that stage 1–3 patients are not on the non-nephrologists' radar screens.[68] The Mayo nephrologists rely on the PCP to screen for CKD and its risk factors and to treat comorbidities and CV risk factors. There is overlap even once a patient is in the CKD clinic; however, the nephrologist naturally takes over more of the care as the disease progresses. There needs to be a better understanding of who does what and when, and communication tools are available to assist with that important task.[69] Importantly, Mayo physicians are salaried, so relations between physicians are not determined by economic considerations, unlike the situation in most practice settings outside of a staff model or academic organization.

In the Mayo system, therefore, there is an intense focus on education of PCPs and patients. A key realization by the Mayo nephrologists has been that other specialists read only their own literature and go to their own meetings, which requires that CKD research results be published in specialty-relevant journals and presented at specialty meetings. In addition, the nephrologists encouraged Mayo to report eGFRs for all serum creatinine lab test determinations, which created some concern on the part of non-nephrologists, particularly because of the high prevalence of abnormal values in patients over 70 years of age.[70] Patients who come from outside referrals, and their physicians, are educated about CKD on an individual basis. There are also education classes—both basic and advanced—for patients in the CKD clinic, which are led by one of the NPs and include a dietitian and a social worker who also serve the dialysis clinic.

Clinic Procedures

All patients enter the Mayo Clinic through the central appointments desk. Renal patients proceed to Mayo nephrology for initial consultation. If appropriate, they will be referred subsequently to the CKD clinic. However, given the complex nature of Mayo as a referral center, not all CKD patients are seen in the CKD clinic. Patient wait time for an initial appointment is priority-based following a determination of need and urgency.

Diagnosis involves estimating GFR using an equation developed by the MDRD clinical trial and/or measuring 24-hour urine creatinine clearance, as well as occasionally measuring iothalamate clearance. CKD staging is based on eGFR using the MDRD formula. The laboratory used by the CKD clinic routinely calculates eGFR from a serum creatinine–based estimating equation, as does the hospital. Third-party payers, however, do not reimburse for eGFR if billed separately and derived from a creatinine-based equation.

Patients present with a variety of symptoms, as in most nephrology practices. Some patients present for consultation only; these patients are referred mainly by PCPs but sometimes by specialists, account for perhaps 40 percent of the CKD patients, and are seen once or twice. The practice consists mostly of stage 3 or 4 patients referred by PCPs, family care physicians, or internists who will be seen initially by a nephrologist and then seen every 3–6 months on an ongoing basis, depending on stage and stability; these patients account for about 50–60 percent of all CKD patients. Then, from this group, patients are recruited into the CKD clinic. According to Dr. Haley, "Most but not all patients are interested in the multidisciplinary clinic approach, and dropouts are rare." Both the nephrologist and the NP see each patient on each visit; the nephrologist assesses progress on goals of care and stability of kidney function and makes decisions on medications, diet, activity, needed tests, procedures, consultation, and the next visit interval. He or she completes the standard electronic medical record (EMR), Power-Notes, which captures discrete quality goal-based data as well as the elements required for adequate documentation. The NPs keep in touch with the patients between visits, help manage scheduling, and see that the tests ordered are received, in addition to interim protocol-based visits with a subset of patients for anemia and hypertension management.

Each nephrologist takes care of his or her own patients, and this increases patient satisfaction, a major driver for the Mayo nephrologists. Patients are more likely to follow advice and instructions—e.g., are more likely to have an AV fistula created in preparation for ESRD—if they are comfortable with and know the physician and NP. An AV fistula takes perhaps eight weeks to develop before it can be used effectively. If dialysis is required before a fistula is mature and another vascular access method is needed, patient mortality is higher.

By stage 4, patients are also being seen by a dietitian. In addition, vascular surgeons manage a vascular access program. Although they are peripheral to and not within the clinic, there is a monthly vascular conference focused on presentations of patients with access problems. The NPs coordinate all of this.

Overall, the advantages of the CKD clinic include seeing patients on a timely basis, managing the many aspects of optimal management in a standardized way, and making the most efficient use of clinic organization and PowerNotes.

Health Information Technology System

The CKD clinic uses PowerNotes, a function of its EMR system, which allows it to collect a set of relevant, discrete, standardized data at each visit. In addition, all CKD clinic patients are entered into a database designed by Mayo staff (StudyTrax), which allows the clinic to track outcomes such as mortality, hospitalizations, patient satisfaction, anemia, and blood pressure control.

The nephrology PowerNotes were developed in late 2002. A templated visit note is incorporated in the medical record; patient data are imported directly from the EMR to the note, which includes the various domains of CKD care: blood pressure, hematology (hemoglobin, iron, ferritin), kidney function (the laboratory estimate of GFR), mineral metabolism, and nutrition. Follow-up is also part of the electronic system. Visit data can be documented very quickly, without transcription, and are immediately available. KDOQI and RPA guideline values and recommendations are embedded in the CKD domains of the PowerNotes to provide reminders to address goals of care at the time of each visit. Access to this data system is available to everyone at Mayo who has access to the EMR, including the hospital environment. The database enables the group to follow the CKD patient cohort prospectively, aggregate and analyze data, and provide feedback reports on quality metrics.

Practice Guidelines

The Mayo CKD clinic uses clinical practice guidelines, which are embedded in its data system.[71, 72] It uses the field-tested RPA advanced CKD Management Toolkit Clinical Practice Measures (CPMs) for blood pressure, ACE inhibitor or ARB therapy, anemia care, mineral metabolism, metabolic acidosis, lipids, nutrition (albumin, body weight), timing of renal replacement therapy preparation (discussion of modality, referral for AV fistula, transplant), counseling and rehabilitation, and influenza vaccination.[73] This HIT system facilitates systematic care, adherence to guideline-based checklists, and effective management of joint doctor-nurse relations.

The RPA task force led by Dr. Haley developed a CKD toolkit, which in his judgment has been well received:

> It has led to improved processes of care, but it has only been in use since 2005, so we don't yet have evidence on outcomes of care. [However,] it has helped with patient satisfaction, and it has helped in engaging allied health professionals. Users of the toolkit believe that it improves outcomes.

Many of Haley's patients like the "diary" tool—a "report card" to the patient, which allows them to keep up with their numbers as well as their medications. The diary is a visual tool that explains the goals of care in lay terms, e.g., why diet is important. It is used both for one-time and ongoing activities.

External Relations

Two aspects of major importance that are external to most CKD clinics are reimbursement and relations between CKD clinics and the large dialysis chains. Only the first of these pertains to the Mayo CKD clinic.

Reimbursement

Private health insurers, in the view of the Mayo nephrologists, need to react prospectively to CKD, but so far this is not happening. The value of the CKD clinic in slowing progression to ESRD and offsetting future costs should be apparent to payers, but because exposure to risk may be relatively short (patients frequently come and go in health plans), they are unlikely to see this as a long-term commitment and payoff. The dilemma also is that the less-well-insured often turn out to be the more needy.

Both Medicaid and Medicare reimburse at a level that fails to adequately pay for the time and resource-intensive care that these patients need. Thus, most nephrology practices lose money in the office on CKD care, including the group at Mayo. This negative incentive to provide optimal CKD management results in what we have now—increasing numbers of patients progressing to ESRD in poor condition, imposing a high personal and societal burden.

Future Challenges

To the Mayo group, there are at least three significant barriers to the provision of high-quality CKD care. The first is the lack of knowledge and understanding on the part of non-nephrologists of the need to screen patients at risk for CKD and to refer appropriately. The second is the lack of time available to the nephrologist who is required to review and address the multiple complex issues surrounding optimal care for each patient. Finally, some patients' lack of ability to comply with evidence-based advice and treatment is a significant barrier, some of which is due to financial or other socioeconomic factors, some to lack of adequate caregiver support, and some to lifestyle choices.

There are other challenges to the successful implementation of the Mayo CKD practice and, by extension, to the country. First, the CKD population continues to grow. Second, the demand for nephrologists to provide CKD care has already outstripped the supply of nephrologists. Thus, as a general nephrology practice grows, so does the number of CKD patients needing follow-up care, creating a situation of concern with respect to quality, service, and safety.

Although this population of patients faces unique risks, complications, and needs, there is a huge opportunity to improve care and outcomes. However, payers are demanding results, not just visit time. Health services research is needed to determine the impact of CKD guidelines, measures, and CKD clinics on outcomes including mortality, CV events, progression to end-stage kidney failure, hospitalizations, and quality of life.

To summarize, Dr. Haley identified the following drivers of CKD care as it develops in the near future (see Box 5.1). The factors affecting such care are not all consistent with each other. Indeed, the resource limitations, including an insufficient supply of nephrologists and poor reimbursement, suggest that progress in CKD care lies well beyond the control of physicians at the local clinic or practice.

Box 5.1: Drivers of Chronic Kidney Disease Care

- Increasing demand for nephrology services versus limited time and resources
- Special population: unique CKD-related risks, complications, needs
- Evidence of suboptimal, highly variable care
- Existence of guidelines and measures for optimal care
- Poor reimbursement for CKD care
- Need for efficient care model that adds value
- Need for quality measurement system

CHAPTER SIX

Indiana Medical Associates, Fort Wayne, Indiana

Richard A. Rettig, Ph.D.;* Stephen McMurray, M.D.; Roberto B. Vargas, M.D., M.P.H.;
and Allen R. Nissenson, M.D.

Indiana Medical Associates (IMA) is a multispecialty physician group with several offices and dialysis centers operating in a 70-mile radius covering northeast Indiana and parts of Ohio. Its main office is in Fort Wayne, Indiana. The CKD practice developed in the late 1990s during a time when growth in the number of incident dialysis patients in the region began to level off, and the shift from ESRD care began to move toward outpatient care while occurrences of diabetes-related CKD began to increase. Development of a CKD focus began before the development of CKD guidelines, but IMA now incorporates both KDOQI and RPA guidelines in its protocols. IMA does not have a CKD "clinic" but is more of an organized nephrology practice group with cardiologists as the primary referral base. Referrals are based on clinical criteria of renal function and anemia, and CKD care is focused on stage 3 and 4 patients. The group currently uses a disease management system that combines guidelines with an IT data system. Observational data suggest that these changes have resulted in improved fistula placement, dialysis training, and anemia management. Future concerns include uncertainty over the ability to cross-subsidize CKD care as dialysis care reimbursement evolves, as well as the role of CKD care in relation to the influence of large dialysis organizations.

Practice Overview

IMA is a 34-physician group practice that includes ten nephrologists. The group is located on the southwest side of Fort Wayne, Indiana, on the campus of the Lutheran Medical Center. Lutheran Hospital, with approximately 400 beds, is the largest hospital in the city and has satellite hospitals in Warsaw, Indiana, and Peru, Indiana. Stephen McMurray, M.D., a past president of the IMA group and its principal spokesman, has been with the practice for 30 years.

IMA operates in northeast Indiana, a region with a population base of 1.2 million, which includes Fort Wayne (with a population of 200,000) as well as all of northeast Indiana and part of northwest Ohio. IMA provides tertiary care for kidney disease for northeast Indiana from its Fort Wayne base of operations. IMA has three main offices, but its nephrologists visit clinics at nine satellite centers and nine dialysis clinics to see CKD patients. The Indiana locations include Warsaw, Marion, Wabash, Auburn, and Huntington; the Ohio locations are Van Wert, Bryan, Defiance, and Paulding.

---

* This case study is based on a site visit interview conducted by Dr. Rettig on September 11, 2007, supplemented by several PowerPoint presentations by Dr. McMurray; it was preceded by a telephone interview conducted by Dr. Rettig with Dr. McMurray on April 6, 2006.

Origins and Development of Practice

The forerunner of today's IMA practice was begun in 1973. In 1977, Fort Wayne Nephrology was spun off from the internal medicine group but remained closely affiliated. Later, several subspecialty groups formed Indiana Regional Medical Consultants, which evolved into IMA. The practice included the specialties of endocrinology, pulmonology, gastroenterology, nephrology, and internal medicine.

In 1977, the practice had 42 dialysis patients; by 1996, it had 323 dialysis patients; and today it has 560 dialysis patients at its multiple dialysis sites across northeast Indiana and northwest Ohio. Inpatients were initially treated at Old Lutheran (the downtown site of Lutheran Hospital, which was subsequently closed when a new facility was built), but as the practice grew, its nephrologists saw patients at all the Fort Wayne hospitals.

The nephrology practice of IMA has evolved from a practice that initially focused on intensive care medicine, including coordination of critical care services for the medical providers of dialysis services, as well as an office practice. IMA now provides in-hospital nephrology consultative services, with fewer critical care services. The dialysis and medical director activities now account for much more of the practice time. The office practice and the provision of CKD care have expanded significantly over the last 10 years.

From 1996 to 2006, IMA was affiliated with the Renal Care Group (RCG), a proprietary large dialysis organization. FMC purchased RCG in April 2006, and IMA has been affiliated with FMC since then. A venture arm of the practice, Indiana Dialysis Management, participates in a vascular access center, manages medical director contracts with the dialysis units, and engages in joint ventures with dialysis organizations.

IMA's CKD practice developed in the late 1990s, due partly to the slowing of the growth in the Indiana incident dialysis population from 7 percent per year to 1 or 2 percent. Given that each new dialysis patient represented $5,000–$6,000 in yearly physician revenue, it had been easy in the time of growth to determine when to add a new physician to the practice. When the growth of the Indiana dialysis population slowed, questions arose about how IMA could continue to grow its dialysis population and the associated physician revenue. IMA focused on improving outcomes throughout the continuum of CKD, with the goal of reducing 90-day patient mortality and morbidity and improving the care of those progressing to dialysis. During the 1990s, there was a shift in care of the ESRD patient from an inpatient to an outpatient focus. This resulted in the practice seeing fewer patients in the hospital and more in the dialysis facilities and the office. The practice shifts described above led to a change in the distribution of income sources.

There was also a change in the conditions found among the patient population, from a preponderance of hypertension, glomerulonephritis, and polycystic kidney disease as the leading causes of CKD to diabetes as the primary cause of renal failure. Diabetes now accounts for 50 percent of all of IMA's ESRD patients and over one-half of its stage 3 and 4 CKD patients.

IMA has been the site of several pilot projects to improve the care of CKD and ESRD patients. In 2003, Amgen asked RCG to develop a CKD model that a practice could replicate. This included developing a practice and business model of a CKD program. RCG contracted with IMA to develop the program, which also involved six other practices affiliated with RCG. Similarly, IMA nephrology developed a program focused on diabetes care in dialysis to demonstrate that care of the diabetic patient in the dialysis unit could be improved.[74]

The Indiana Medical Associates Chronic Kidney Disease Practice

CKD clinics and practices are in an early stage of development. They are engaged simultaneously in developing clinical routines and protocols, creating internal organizational processes, and establishing external relationships with those on whom they depend for patient referrals and payment for services. In this regard, they are unlike well-established clinical practices with a predictable inflow of patients, which have a range of relatively well-understood diseases for which there exist clinical procedures that are reimbursable (and reimbursed) by health insurers.

The Patient Population

The IMA patient population is 60 percent male and 40 percent female, with an average age of 69.6 years. In 2006,

- 60 percent of patients had an initial diagnosis of stage 3–5 CKD.
- 50 percent of patients were diagnosed with diabetes mellitus as the primary cause of CKD.
- 82 percent of patients had Medicare, 3 percent had Medicaid, and the rest had private insurance.

The practice does not trace the ethnicity of its patients. Currently, there are over 1,200 patients in the IMA CKD database.

IMA sees 85 percent of CKD patients before dialysis is initiated. Among the problems of treating CKD patients identified by IMA is the need to get the appropriate balance between enough of the right patients and not too many of the wrong patients, i.e., those with normal renal function and microalbuminuria who would be more appropriately treated by the PCP.

The more impoverished patients, perhaps 15 percent of the total, are typically seen in the emergency room. Clinic leadership felt that these patients were about evenly split between minority and nonminority patients. Over time, an increase has occurred in the local Hispanic population, and IMA is just beginning to see an increase in the number of Hispanic patients.

Outreach, Education, and Referrals

Central to the viability of any CKD clinic is a steady flow of patients. Consequently, outreach and educational activities are as integral to CKD clinics and practices as are the clinical procedures used to treat patients.

IMA has not established a CKD *clinic* but has organized a *practice*. In most practice settings, doctors do not make referrals to clinics but to other doctors. For IMA, cardiologists and cardiac surgeons are the single biggest source of referrals of CKD patients. Referrals also come from endocrinologists, PCPs, and family practitioners. However, these physicians, who provide perhaps 40 percent of the total patient referrals, are each usually responsible for referring only one or two patients to a nephrologist.

CKD educational efforts are carried out by IMA nephrologists in various medical offices of PCPs and cardiologists. In addition, nurse practitioners are used to spread the word about treatment options. IMA has a reasonable flow of patients. However, there is competition, and IMA gets only 70 percent of the ESRD patients in the local geographic area.

Practice Organization

The IMA group practice includes 34 physicians. Ten of these are nephrologists, including one transplant nephrologist. Two of the nephrologists are part-time, and the remaining eight are full-time in the practice. There are also three physician extenders (two NPs and one PA).

The IMA contract with RCG to develop a CKD model was to include these clinical criteria for CKD patients: a creatinine level greater than 2 mg/dL, a creatinine clearance less than 30 mL/min., and a need for anemia management. An important component of the model was the use of data, including clinical pathways, for anemia, diabetes, dialysis orientation, vascular access, lipid management, bone metabolism, and vaccination. IMA then educated the nursing staff and implemented the model using data and pathways over a five-year period.

Health Information Technology Systems

IMA has used multiple HIT systems. In the dialysis clinics, the initial dialysis HIT system involved an electronic medical record known as Renal Star, which was adopted in 1992 and was designed to collect data regarding dialysis patients in the clinics, as well as to provide a billing function. This was IMA's first foray into an EMR. Around 2000, the dialysis clinics switched to the RCG AMI system, a commercial database system, which evolved into an excellent EMR with robust data extraction capability. The practice uses the EMR and available outcomes data to drive improvements in clinical care in the dialysis clinic.

A separate program was developed to perform an initial risk assessment of the dialysis population, with the goal of identifying those patients with significant comorbidities at the start of dialysis. This evolved into a dialysis case management system under RCG and was used for diabetes care management. The same system was then adapted to collect data for the CKD population.

In the office practice, IMA developed a paper CKD data collection system in the mid-1990s, which was used until 2002. At that time, IMA implemented an RCG CKD data tracking system, which was used until 2006. IMA was able to track the CKD population, review outcomes, and generate exception reports identifying those patients who needed interventions (e.g., a pneumovax immunization). The practice implemented an EMR at the start of 2007, and the prior CKD data tracking system was discontinued. This was done in anticipation of pay-for-performance to allow for better data sharing without the group and with outside entities.

Currently, the data extraction capabilities of the EMR are limited and have slowed IMA's ability to collect and analyze CKD results, but these areas are expected to improve in the near future. Underlying the above efforts is the conviction of the IMA practice that an effective HIT system is essential to manage a CKD practice and achieve the desired results.

Clinic Procedures

Initial patient wait time for an evaluation is 4–6 weeks. The frequency of patient visits is driven by patient needs and characteristics, which vary from monthly to quarterly, depending on CKD stage and management program. On average, patients are seen every 2–3 months. The practice has no dedicated dietitian.

IMA's CKD treatment focuses on stages 3 and 4, and its clinical pathways are designed to address these stages. There is no organized clinical pathway for stage 2 CKD. Regarding staging, most northeast Indiana laboratories calculate eGFR. The IMA office laboratory calculates eGFR as well. However, no statewide requirement exists for calculating eGFR, and third-party payers do not pay for eGFRs.

IMA has confirmed what has been published in many studies: that eGFR is highly variable. The availability of a measurement that consistently approaches sensitivity and specificity of inulin clearance (the gold standard for assessing kidney function) across the entire range of kidney function would be highly desirable. The variability of eGFR and the implication of a low eGFR, especially in select populations such as the elderly, can make a big difference in clinical decisionmaking. In an older person, a report of an eGFR of 30 mL/min. could reflect significant underlying renal pathology or nonspecific age-related decline in renal function. That variation in clinical decisionmaking, if relying on eGFR alone, can determine whether or not a patient is referred for dialysis orientation or a fistula placement.[75]

Practice Guidelines

IMA began to develop clinical pathways before the KDOQI guidelines were published. After the KDOQI and RPA guidelines were published, IMA altered its pathways to be consistent with those guidelines. The current guidelines account for local variances. The practice regards guidelines as essential to managing a population of patients but requires consensus about the guidelines by users and a process for data acquisition to measure adherence. At IMA, a physician and nurse interact in implementing the guidelines.

The big challenge for IMA is in changing the culture of practice. None of the nurses had prior training in pathways, and the nephrologists were not initially enthusiastic proponents of the use of guidelines. After considerable education and experience in using the guidelines, physicians and nonphysicians agreed that decreasing variation in practice was a desirable goal and that the guidelines were effective tools to enable this, with appropriate support from a robust information system.

In 2002, IMA introduced a practice-based CKD disease management system that incorporated clinical practice guidelines and utilized a then-adequate HIT data system.[76] The system focused on anemia management (including administration of Aranesp) of CKD patients, but clinical pathways were also developed for dialysis modality education, AV fistula placement, osteodystrophy management, lipid management, blood pressure monitoring, and vaccinations (for pneumococcal pneumonia, hepatitis B, and influenza).

What were the effects of this 15-month disease management effort? IMA reports that it saw

- a reduction in the prevalence of anemia
- an increase in the percentage of patients who achieved hemoglobin above 11 g/dL with Aranesp from 60 percent to 74 percent
- an increase in the number of CKD patients starting dialysis with hemoglobin greater than 10 g/dL from 61 percent to 74 percent, in a geographic region where fewer than half the patients starting dialysis before 2002 had hemoglobin above 10 g/dL
- an increase in dialysis modality training from 54 percent to 80 percent
- an increase in AV fistula placement in patients with CrCl below 30 mL/min. from 46 percent to 54 percent
- a decrease in first 90-day mortality among CKD patients starting dialysis from 10 percent to 6 percent.[77]

External Relations

Two aspects of major importance external to the clinic are reimbursement and relations between CKD clinics and the large dialysis chains.

Reimbursement

The IMA experience makes clear that the care of CKD patients requires cross-subsidy from some other reimbursed source. The two sources that have financed CKD care in this case have been Medicare payments for the treatment of dialysis patients and Medicare reimbursement for erythropoietin (Aranesp, in this instance). However, the former has been under continued pressure over many years and no longer provides a financial base for CKD care. And the latter has been under more immediate pressure because of recent controversy over appropriate hemoglobin target levels.[78] For example, excess revenue on Aranesp has been cross-subsidizing CKD care, but that revenue stream has diminished considerably.

IMA belies that CMS could facilitate the provision of optimal CKD care by nephrologists by

1. paying a CKD management fee
2. allowing some dollars to be returned to good performers under pay for performance
3. commingling Part A and Part B Medicare funds.

Large Dialysis Organizations

A major issue regarding CKD care involves the relationship between an individual clinic or practice to the large dialysis organizations. IMA has been part of two large dialysis organizations: From 1996 to 2006, it was affiliated with RCG; since the purchase of RCG by FMC in April 2006, it has been affiliated with FMC.

RCG began the process of indentifying practices that were involved in CKD care and has improved the CKD information system. FMC has embraced the CKD process and is encouraging practices to enhance and develop their CKD programs.

CHAPTER SEVEN

St. Clair Specialty Physicians, P.C., Detroit, Michigan

Richard A. Rettig, Ph.D.;* Robert Provenzano, M.D.; Roberto B. Vargas, M.D., M.P.H.;
and Allen R. Nissenson, M.D.

St. Clair Specialty Physicians is an urban nephrology practice located in a single facility in Detroit, Michigan. In 1988, the practice began to focus on CKD because of the high number of patients presenting with "early renal insufficiency." The practice's principal referral source is community physicians. Roughly 60 percent of patients have diabetes and 40 percent have hypertension in this largely African-American patient population. St. Clair is an integrated physician practice, which includes generalist physicians, nephrologists, a transplant physician, and surgeons. Clinical NPs coordinate care and staff, and there is external physician comanagement with cardiologists. In addition, the practice has community outreach programs in conjunction with local civic groups, nonprofit organizations, and media outlets. CKD care includes patients from stages 1–5; stage identification is facilitated by a state Medicaid policy requiring automated eGFR calculations from serum creatinines. Care is guided by protocols and implemented by multidisciplinary teams. The practice does not have registered dieticians, social workers, or other nonreimbursed service providers on staff. Future challenges include the need to align financial incentives and to help insurers and referring physicians understand the importance of early identification referral. They also identified the need for greater attention to address disparities in access to care for minority and underserved populations.

Practice Overview

St. Clair Specialty Physicians, P.C., a CKD practice, is an independent entity physically housed in St. John Hospital and Medical Center's Professional Services Building. St. John Hospital and Medical Center is a teaching hospital affiliated with the Wayne State University School of Medicine. It is located in Detroit, Michigan, near the boundary of Detroit and Grosse Pointe. The clinic draws its patients from southeast Michigan, including all of greater Detroit and its suburbs. The current chief operating officer is Robert Provenzano, M.D.

---

* This case study is based on an extended site visit interview conducted by Dr. Rettig on April 18, 2007, supplemented by later correspondence; it had been preceded by a telephone survey interview conducted by Dr. Rettig on April 13, 2006.

Origins and Development

St. Clair Specialty Physicians, P.C., was formed in 1988 from an existing practice. St. Clair's focus went beyond just ESRD care to include the care of CKD patients, which in this period was also called the care of patients with "early renal insufficiency."

What prompted the reorientation toward CKD? More and more patients were presenting with varying degrees of kidney disease, not all of which were end-stage. Although it was known that the disease was progressive, there were no early data demonstrating that the course of the CKD was modifiable. However, therapies and medications were becoming available that could slow progression to kidney failure, beginning with ACE inhibitors and followed by oral vitamin D. The practice was also interested in increasing the efficiency of dialysis facilities because ESRD treatment funding was sufficient to cross-subsidize CKD care; efficiencies in the former made support for the latter possible.

The strategy of the St. Clair CKD practice was (and remains), first, to identify the at-risk population and offer treatment. If a patient has kidney disease, the objective is to determine whether the disease is reversible. If it is, the practice treats the CKD. If not, treatment is initiated to forestall progression. If CKD cannot be reversed despite therapy, or if CKD is identified too late for reasonable intervention, patients are prepared for renal replacement therapy, either dialysis or, if appropriate, kidney transplantation.

The practice was created to provide a community service. African-Americans were disproportionately represented among CKD patients. The business model for St. Clair encompassed the entire cadre of CKD patients and ESRD patients, as well as all related conditions, by providing an integrated, stratified system of care specifically focused on these unique patients' needs. If this approach was successful, it was hoped that health care providers, health insurers, and health plans would refer more patients to the practice. At the time, such patients tended not to stay enrolled in a single plan for long, and, therefore, initiation of intensive, and often expensive, therapy was not in the fiscal interests of the health plans. In addition, ESRD patients were only a very small number of their total enrollees.

When these efforts were initiated in 1988, there were few practices focused on CKD. Most of the nephrology specialty was focused on ESRD care. Even the state chapter of the NKF showed little interest in CKD at that time. To fund the care of CKD patients, the practice purchased half the hospital dialysis business and entered a joint venture called the St. John Dialysis Network. In four years, the dialysis program grew from 76 patients to 900 patients, and the profits funded the expansion of the CKD program. Over the next several years, the practice partnered with several large dialysis organizations to benefit from the significant economies of scale that such a relationship provided. The joint venture relationship included ESRD, CKD, and vascular access centers.

The St. Clair Chronic Kidney Disease Practice

St. Clair is a completely integrated CKD practice, with outreach, education, and patient referrals integral to a clinic that provides comprehensive clinical services for stage 3, stage 4, and stage 5 CKD patients. The clinic is run by NPs but supervised by nephrologists. It includes a vascular surgeon and two vascular access centers; a transplant team (surgeons as well as transplant nephrologists); a primary care unit (staffed by internal medicine physicians); a research unit; conventional, nocturnal and home hemodialysis modalities; and a unit devoted to peritoneal dialysis (CAPD/CCPD).

The Patient Population

The St. Clair CKD patient population has grown substantially in recent years, more than doubling from 2000 to 2006, as shown in Table 7.1. In 2006, diabetes accounted for 58 percent of the St. Clair CKD patients, and hypertension accounted for 40 percent. Seventy to eighty percent of the patients are African-American; of these, 15 percent are 25 years old or younger, 5–6 percent are over 85, 30 percent are in the 65–84 age group, another 30 percent are in the 55–64 age group, and the balance are in the 25–44 age group.

There are striking differences in both the incidence and prevalence of CKD between African-American and Caucasian patients, which is of concern to the practice. It remains all too common for the practice to have first-degree relatives in the same dialysis facilities. In one facility, the practice has a mother, a daughter, and an uncle. Not only are the incidence

Table 7.1
The St. Clair Patient Population, by Office (2000–2006)

	2000	2001	2002	2003	2004	2005	2006
Detroit							
New	430	445	567	620	659	603	954
Follow-up	3,892	4,401	4,989	6,004	5,939	6,112	9,432
Shelby							
New		98	121	155	169	217	284
Follow-up		786	1,002	1,612	1,002	1,039	1,838
Warren							
New			56	67	103	120	165
Follow-up			555	789	1,225	1,326	1,817
Grosse Pointe							
New							41
Follow-up							400
Riverview							
New						34	65
Follow-up						276	766
Farmington Hill							
New							155
Follow-up							1,435
Totals							
New	430	543	744	842	931	974	1,664
Follow-up	3,892	5,187	6,546	8,405	8,166	8,753	15,688

and prevalence of CKD and ESRD much greater among minority populations, but, with the exception of dialysis, the underlying health problems of these populations are typically going untreated from one generation to the next.

Outreach, Education, and Referrals

Community outreach seeks to identify patients and provides educational activities directed to individuals, families, community groups, and the relevant physicians in the community. For example, the clinic works with African-American churches and community groups, such as the Rotary Clubs, to emphasize the personal responsibility of individuals in taking care of their health and in seeking a physician. Representatives of the clinic go to local events at nursing homes, which have become very sophisticated about educating their residents on health care. In addition, St. Clair staff visit high schools in conjunction with the NKF of Michigan. They also go to women's hair salons and educate stylists about CKD, as a way to reach the African-American community; the practice has also extended this approach to men's barbershops.

Education about CKD takes various forms. St. Clair has established relations with local community newspapers, publishes health stories on vascular disease and related subjects, and has partnered with local television stations on educational initiatives.

A major focus of the clinic is on referrals from physicians treating patients at risk for CKD. The principal patient referral sources for the clinic are PCPs (family practitioners, internists), who provide 70 percent of referrals; the remaining 30 percent come from cardiologists and endocrinologists.

For early-stage CKD (stages 1 and 2), St. Clair focuses on educating PCPs and the community about CKD, especially the at-risk population groups, such as hypertensive individuals, diabetics, African-Americans, and those with a first-degree relative with kidney disease. The education involves a physician or an NP giving a presentation on high blood pressure and its complications, for example.

For late-stage CKD (stages 3, 4, and 5), St. Clair engages in intensified efforts to inform the local community about the value of its approach. St. Clair educates the resident physicians and fellows at St. John Hospital, which is an academic teaching hospital. St. Clair also seeks to educate PCPs; an NP might make a presentation at a luncheon or a dinner. The education of cardiologists is very specific and focuses on reducing patient length of stay associated with acute renal failure (often caused by intravenous contrast dye), thus increasing hospital revenue. Forty percent of cardiac patients have CKD, a fact that is mostly unknown to both patients and their physicians. For endocrinologists, the clinic offers the opportunity to offload difficult patients and avoid having to treat CKD.

The need for the comanagement of CKD patients emerges from the relations between CKD physicians (nephrologists) and the other physicians treating the patient. Traditionally, comanagement has meant giving up care of a patient only at the point of the need for dialysis, not at CKD stage 3 or 4. Given the fragmentation of care in the U.S. health care system, relations with the other medical specialties are often predicated on dollars. The PCPs have some fears that their patients will be taken away or that they will lose money. They also often think that there is little or nothing that nephrologists can do that is unique or that the PCPs could not do themselves.

St. Clair staff feel that, in order for patient referrals to occur as they should, the financial barriers that interfere with patient referral should be removed. What is needed, in the view of the practice, are mechanisms that would *require* a patient to be seen by a nephrologist once

CKD is identified. Although this approach may sound self-serving, there are many precedents for this approach in hospitals: Patients with cardiovascular disease or coronary artery disease are routinely referred to cardiologists, and HIV/AIDS patients to infectious disease physicians.

Stage 5 CKD patients are the clear purview of nephrologists. These patients are high-risk, require anemia therapy, have vascular access issues, and need intense education about transplantation and dialysis. However, one barrier to providing CKD care in southeastern Michigan, as elsewhere in the country, is that many nephrologists resist providing such care, as reimbursement focuses so strongly on ESRD treatment.

Institutional relations also influence referrals with hospitals or other institutions with dialysis units. At the time of this study, in mid-2007, St. Clair was in the process of concluding merger talks with nephrology practices in the major population areas of Flint, Port Huron, Grand Rapids, and Marquette. In general, most of these practices have relied heavily on income generated from dialysis patients. As the practice begins to give more emphasis to CKD and other ancillary aspects of nephrology, the benefits of merging with larger practices become clear. Efficiencies in purchasing, billing, and other aspects of practice infrastructure become attractive.

Health Information Technology System

St. Clair designed its own HIT system. The system is an asset that St. Clair uses for internal management—billing, auditing, clinical practice guidelines, patient records, treatment quality, and outcomes—and for external marketing of its business.

Clinic Procedures

Staging of CKD patients is done using the MDRD equation to calculate eGFR. The clinic laboratory calculates eGFR routinely whenever a serum creatinine is obtained. Legislation passed in Michigan in 2004 requires all laboratories doing business with the state Medicaid program to provide eGFR calculations any time a serum creatinine is ordered. Although limited to a state program, the requirement effectively applies to all care, as laboratories cannot easily differentiate between Medicaid and non-Medicaid patients. Michigan legislators hoped that this requirement would result in earlier identification and referral of at-risk patients (13 states now have this or a similar requirement).

Once a patient is referred to the CKD clinic, care is guideline-directed. An advanced practice nurse (APN) follows a formal intake procedure for identified patients. The patient then sees a nephrologist, who provides a formal consult resulting in a diagnosis, staging, and placement in an appropriate guideline-directed program of care. Anemia management, hypertension, bone disease, and vascular access evaluation are provided utilizing clinical practice guidelines, which are updated annually. The patient is then transferred back to the APN (or to a PA), working under the supervision of a nephrologist, who provides follow-up CKD management.

The wait time for a new patient appointment is 24 hours. This is an open clinic. The nephrologists see all new patients, determine whether they have kidney disease, and develop a treatment plan for those patients diagnosed with CKD. The care of CKD patients is then turned over to the clinic. On later visits, the patient is seen by the NPs or PAs. Data collection (e.g., the vitals) is done by the medical assistants. The administration of medications (e.g., Epogen or iron) is done by the RNs.

St. Clair has no dietitian because it is not cost-effective to do so, given the minimal reimbursement available for their services. In the view of the practice, the nutritional aspect of CKD care is a midlevel task that can be done effectively by the NP or PA. The clinic also does not have a social worker, as there is no reimbursement for their services either. Patients are referred to the hospital if a social worker is needed.

Special protocols are applied for the CKD stage 4 and CKD stage 5 patients. Patients are referred to the vascular surgery team for vein mapping, which is done on site. They meet with the vascular surgeon and have an access (i.e., a fistula) placed if they are a candidate for hemodialysis. If a patient is a transplant candidate, he or she is referred to the transplant team.

For stage 5 patients, the CKD clinic begins the transition either to dialysis or transplantation. The vascular surgeons and the transplant physicians are integrated into the CKD clinic. If a transplant is not indicated, the APN will educate the patient about the various dialysis modalities, and the patient will choose based on what best suits his or her quality of life. The prospective dialysis patient will then be vein-mapped and have a fistula inserted or will be tentatively scheduled for peritoneal dialysis catheter placement. If transplant is recommended, the patient is referred to the transplant team for education and preemptive transplantation.

All ancillary services are provided in the clinic; the patient does not have to go anywhere else. Within the St. Clair system there are three primary CKD sites (large clinics that provide all or most services). Each primary clinic has a smaller satellite outreach program in a "hub and spoke" configuration. There are now about 4,000 patients in the St. Clair CKD database.

The experience of the St. Clair clinic, like that of most other clinics, had been that patients were referred to the practice in the very late stages of kidney disease, although since the hospital and the state of Michigan have required calculation of eGFR using the MDRD formula, there have been a significant number of earlier referrals. For underserved populations, however, particularly African-Americans, access to care is limited. Moreover, in the inner city of Detroit, there are a number of "doc in the box" clinics, literally clinics on the corner, where these patients go for general care. At least 15–20 percent of late-stage CKD patients come from these clinics.

Practice Guidelines

The practice has used the NKF and RPA CKD toolkits but has found the latter to be more user friendly, although it focuses only on stages 3, 4, and 5. The RPA CKD toolkit has been field-tested, which has already led to refinements; it is now being field-tested for the second time following modifications.

St. Clair also uses clinical performance measures (CPMs) to track the care of its CKD patients, although there is no reimbursement for doing so. Participating nephrologists receive reports on their performance on these CPMs, which are used as quality improvement tools.

External Relations

Reimbursement

Without question, the most significant barrier that confronts the St. Clair CKD practice is financial. In the words of Dr. Provenzano: "Unfortunately, there are no financial rewards for the efficient provision of quality care in the outpatient setting [Medicare Part B]. The doctors make more money dialyzing patients than preventing the progression of kidney disease." In his view, CMS needs to start evaluating different patients differently: "It is not the case that a patient is a patient is a patient, or that a 15-minute visit is a visit," he said.

The practice is concerned about the CMS focus on ESRD and is convinced that CMS should develop comprehensive care models that reflect that patients could add life years of value through comprehensive, coordinated CKD care. In addition, the practice believes that Congress should target CKD and its comorbidities with the same intensity as it does breast cancer, cardiovascular disease, HIV/AIDS, and lung disease. Appropriate reimbursement is needed for physicians who offer care in integrated, comprehensive CKD clinics that provide "one-stop shopping" and lead to better clinical outcomes.

Currently, CKD care has to be cross-subsidized from the better-reimbursed aspects of care (e.g., ancillaries). Reimbursement is needed in such key areas as patient education and interaction with social workers and dietitians. In addition, many CKD patients do not have insurance and cannot afford necessary, but costly, medications. Staff are stressed by the need to get medications for patients, which can interfere with patient care.

Future Challenges

The benefit of the St. Clair CKD practice to the community consists in identifying people at risk for CKD and offering them treatment and care, which, it is hoped, will have a positive effect on patients' disease processes and, therefore, their lives. Referring physicians benefit from being offered a service that provides expert focused care to their patients and predictable treatment modalities with measurable and reportable outcomes. Hospitals and health care systems benefit by having this population "managed," which decreases inappropriate admissions and length of stay for hospitalized patients. Patients, hospital administrators, nurses, and referring physicians all benefit by the education that the practice offers as it pertains to the CKD and ESRD populations.

Substantial disparities in CKD incidence and prevalence exist between minority and nonminority populations—disparities that extend into the ESRD dialysis population. As a large practice in Detroit with a large underserved minority population, the practice has had to grapple with many questions in this regard, including the questions of what needs to be done to reduce disparities and what needs to be done to provide CKD treatment at the same level as ESRD treatment. Some approaches that have been developed to reduce disparities include:

- Getting doctors to the minority populations. More could be done by applying free market methodologies, such as tax breaks in empowerment zones, and innovative reimbursement strategies to influence care.
- Paying to educate minorities and their extended support systems about CKD. In the local community, more public service educational processes are needed.
- Encouraging private health insurers to mine their databases for CKD patients so that early interventions can be applied.

Winthrop University Hospital, Division of Nephrology and Hypertension, Mineola, Long Island, New York

Richard A. Rettig, Ph.D.;* Stephen Fishbane, M.D.; Roberto B. Vargas, M.D., M.P.H.; and Allen R. Nissenson, M.D.

The Winthrop University Hospital nephrology service is a wholly owned entity of the hospital, located in Mineola, New York, which serves a region of Long Island with a wide range of racial and economic diversity. The nephrology practice is within a teaching hospital with clinical fellow trainees. Interest in transitioning to CKD care was prompted by a sentinel case of delayed referral in the 1990s, which led to outreach lectures and one-on-one visits to PCPs to encourage earlier referrals. Initial practice changes included development of a disease registry, training of the practice nurse to provide patient education, and a "debriefing" of patients on what they have learned immediately after their physician visits. A nurse case manager, who reviews medical records for outliers, also calculates eGFRs and develops individual treatment plans and coordinates care based on patient educational needs. However, additional multidisciplinary resources, such as dieticians, are limited for patients with CKD who are not on dialysis. Encouragingly, state funding for regional health improvement organizations may help foster the development of programs for improved referral and comanagement with PCPs. Challenges for the practice include addressing the increasing need for multidisciplinary office-based care and its high overhead in the face of increasingly stringent financial reimbursement for inpatient, consultative, and ESRD care.

Practice Overview

The Winthrop University Hospital nephrology service consists of a chain of not-for-profit, hospital-owned dialysis units. The service, the Division of Nephrology and Hypertension, is part of the Department of Medicine of the hospital. Winthrop Dialysis Services, a wholly owned entity of the hospital, owns four outpatient dialysis units and manages one inpatient dialysis unit at each of four different Long Island hospitals. CKD patients are seen in the nephrology office practices associated with these dialysis units.

The nephrology service includes five practicing nephrologists. The chief of the division is Steven Fishbane, M.D., who is also associate chairman of the Department of Medicine and director of dialysis services. There are also four fellows in a nephrology fellowship program.

---

* This case study is based on an extended site visit interview conducted by Dr. Rettig on December 11, 2007, and supplemented by later correspondence; the site visit was preceded by a telephone survey interview conducted by Dr. Rettig with Dr. Fishbane on March 28, 2006.

Although nurse practitioners are involved in the dialysis program, none are involved in the office practice.

The geographic area served by Winthrop is centered in Mineola, the county seat of Nassau County, Long Island. The Winthrop nephrology practice serves several communities, with a mix of demographic groups, manifestations of kidney disease, and medical needs. The surrounding communities of Garden City, Westbury, Hempstead, and Uniondale differ in many dimensions, including socioeconomic status, which ranges from very high to poor; race and ethnicity (i.e., the local population includes Caucasians, African-Americans, and Central American immigrants); and presenting condition (i.e., there are many cases of hypertension, diabetes, and obesity, as well as early kidney disease).

Mineola is the main focus of Dr. Fishbane's practice, but he and another nephrologist also practice in Bethpage, 10 miles to the east, where they have a satellite dialysis unit and also see CKD patients. Bethpage has a stable elderly population. Many veterans returned from World War II, settled there, and worked for Northrop Grumman. The population is remarkably homogeneous—many of the patients are 80-year-old white males with heart disease. The task is to address the intersection of kidney disease and heart disease.

Origins and Development of Clinic

Asked how he differentiated CKD care from ESRD, Dr. Fishbane recalled the following:

> The wake-up call for me came in 1995–1996. A second-opinion case came to me, a person with a creatinine of 7.2. The first opinion (from a nephrologist) had been a recommendation of dialysis. A primary care physician had followed this patient for 20 years. Suddenly, with no prior warning, he said to his patient, 'You've got kidney disease and need to see a nephrologist.' The patient later sued the primary care physician for failing to inform him of the emergence of kidney disease. We put him on dialysis and dialyzed him for a couple of years before he died. This set me off. I had read something on early kidney disease, but I began to read more. Jungers and colleagues had written an early paper on the value of nephrology interventions.[79] But this episode was a wake-up call. I started reading about early-stage kidney disease. I went to a meeting in 1998 where Provenzano spoke about this.

Dr. Fishbane wrote a computer program that became the basis of the Winthrop CKD office practice. It generated a report that included basic clinical data, educational information, and blood pressure and creatinine values. "I actually built a calculator," he said, "that predicted the date of kidney failure. I could show a curve of when dialysis would be needed; it would give a specific date."

This "wake-up call" marked the beginning of the practice's outreach efforts on CKD. "In 1996–1997, we did not fully see what was coming," Dr. Fishbane related:

> We brought all the nephrologists in the practice together. My vision was to have a nurse practitioner for the office practice, to create a database, and to introduce a debriefing session after a patient visit. On the database, there were not a lot of guidelines available at that time on hypertension, on anemia. We ended up with a computerized database program that I wrote. But resource constraints limited its development. The debriefing involved a five-minute patient visit with the nurse, who used a checklist of questions after the patient had

seen the physician. We thought that patients were teachable in an encounter with a nurse, which is less stressful that seeing the doctor. The focus was on what the doctor had said, what was discussed about changes in medications, and what illness items were discussed.

The use of the NP did not materialize. Instead, an RN who had been part of the Winthrop peritoneal dialysis practice came on board. Dr. Fishbane described the RN as "high-powered, a strong personality, high competence, strong opinions, who does not hesitate to engage in strong interaction with the docs." The presence of an RN obviated the need for an NP.

"We did understand the trends," Fishbane recalled. "CKD was increasingly recognized, and it carried the need to educate endocrinologists, cardiologists, and primary care physicians. Although CKD was becoming more common in the late 1990s, the NKF KDOQI 2002 guidelines had a huge impact."

The Winthrop Chronic Kidney Disease Practice

The Patient Population

The Winthrop CKD practice does not maintain data concerning its patient population.

Outreach, Education, and Referrals

Dr. Fishbane has given lectures about CKD across Long Island. He lectures about the need for CKD care to PCPs. The major focus of the lectures is creatinine.

Dr. Fishbane has also teamed up with Lionel Mailloux, M.D., a nephrologist at the Northshore Hospital System, who had a strong educational interest and "loves the cardio-renal relationship." The inclusion of a cardiologist increased the effectiveness of the practice team at continuing medical education meetings and other presentations, including dinner talks and lectures. Dr. Fishbane would discuss the value of nephrology intervention, while Dr. Mailloux would discuss cardio-renal function.

In 2002–2006, the team did a lot of outreach to PCPs, including one-on-one meetings and dinners. Dr. Fishbane noted that the doctors have been very receptive to the talks and have begun to acknowledge small decreases in kidney function, leading to earlier referrals.

Dr. Fishbane and his colleagues have also developed other outreach efforts. Long Island is famous for patients having "eight different doctors," according to Fishbane. "The medicalization of people's lives is extensive." Consequently, the Winthrop nephrologists work hard on communication to the referring physicians. They instruct fellows in how to communicate effectively with referring physicians and how to write effective referral letters.

Dr. Fishbane emphasized the importance of his close relationships with cardiologists and related outreach efforts:

Cardiology has made tremendous strides in keeping people alive by cardiac interventions—CABG [coronary artery bypass graft surgery], stents, ACE inhibitors, etc. But at some cost, some heart failure, some kidney disease. This has resulted in a huge change in nephrology in the last 10 years. Consequently, so much depends on how well I work with the cardiologists. We engage in soft comanagement, which requires good communication. The Long Island RHIO [regional health information organization] will help. Half my Bethpage practice involves the comanagement of congestive heart failure.

Clinic Organization

The RN for the Winthrop CKD office practice reviews and comments on the charts for all CKD patients. "She is very effective," Dr. Fishbane noted. "She coordinates the care of the CKD patients, looks at every laboratory result. She does a huge amount of education. She is a brilliant asset for the practice." Winthrop also has an LPN involved in the office practice who follows hemoglobins, makes dose adjustments, and administers EPO and vaccinations.

Clinic Procedures

A patient who enters the Winthrop practice is seen by a nephrologist who makes a full evaluation of his or her medical needs. The patient's GFR will be estimated by the RN or the LPN, who use the NKF website to make the calculation. Treatment plans for the patient are developed, and educational needs are assessed. The nephrologist will decide whether the RN is to be involved for vaccinations, iron, and education. Or he may use a dietitian from the dialysis unit to do a separate sit-down session on diet. "We are sometimes leveraging the dialysis unit," Dr. Fishbane commented.

Two major laboratories serve Long Island. One of those, Quest, calculates eGFR. Dr. Fishbane says that he sometimes gets referrals too early, such as patients with eGFRs in the 60–90 range. "This is especially true for Bethpage; I get early referrals, perhaps too early. If one is going to do screening, develop a treatment plan, etc., then we need a better way to deal with the 60–90 GFR. NKDEP [the National Kidney Disease Education Program] has recognized the problem."

Dr. Fishbane noted that some CKD patients have to wait a long time for an appointment because of a shortage of nephrologists: "A five-month wait [to see a nephrologist] may be an early symptom of things coming apart. It is no answer to say 'add more office access'; we have a shortage of nephrologists, and it's not economically attractive."

Health Information Technology Systems

Initially, Winthrop used Dr. Fishbane's data program to monitor patients, reconcile medications (duplicate use, overuse, misuse), and manage his clinical projects. However, the practice is now moving to an electronic health record. New York state has provided funds for the development of a RHIO, which when operational will allow Winthrop to interact with other hospitals and other doctors; it will connect cardiologists and endocrinologists and will send the medications list and laboratory test results in real time. "We're getting close to implementation," Dr. Fishbane said. "For the future, I can imagine interactions among payers, insurers, primary care physicians."

Practice Guidelines

Winthrop nephrology's CKD practice tends to use the KDOQI guidelines as they are appropriate, but individual physicians use their judgment about each patient. Winthrop tracks outcomes for patients in its half-day teaching clinic. It also provides training for the fellows on blood pressure targets and use of ACE inhibitors. It does not do this in the broader practice, however. It does not have data at this point on blood pressure control or kidney disease progression for individual patients.

External Relations

Reimbursement

Although he did not address reimbursement issues directly, Dr. Fishbane spoke about the economic challenges that the private-practice nephrologist faces:

> All the nephrologists I speak to say that their office practice has exploded in the past five years. But they don't make money there. And for dialysis patients, you are paid for only four visits a month. [A] hospital offers the opportunity for income—consults, acute renal failure, ESRD patients, and practice referrals. The office practice loses money: It has high overhead and reimbursement is not good. So nephrologists squeeze the office time to spend more time in the hospital where the money is. An office practice where you spend 10 minutes per patient, even after a nurse consult, is not the way to go. The question is how to keep oneself available in the hospital and at the same time respond to a growing office practice. A nurse practitioner might see CKD patients initially, and then the doctor sees them the last five minutes of a visit. But the tradeoff hurts: increasing effort in the office versus more time in the hospital, which builds all aspects of the practice.

Winthrop CKD has had some problems because of economic issues. Because of limited staffing, patients typically wait five months for an office appointment. This long wait time sends a mixed message to PCPs: On the one hand, Winthrop encourages referrals; on the other, the practice is typically "too busy" to see referred patients in a timely manner. Options the practice has considered to address this issue include use of more NPs and shorter office visits.

Future Challenges

The major challenge for Winthrop CKD is the growing trend of increased heart failure and its relation to kidney disease. But the question is how to develop systems of care that address the full range of these patients' needs. There are a number of potential approaches for reaching these patients: The number of CKD practices is increasing, as is the number of early-stage CKD patients. More education and outreach to PCPs are needed.

CHAPTER NINE

Conclusions and Recommendations

The recommendations in this chapter focus on both clinical and policy issues to advance the treatment of CKD.

Conclusions

The redefinition of CKD from a late-stage disease, typically requiring dialysis and kidney transplantation, to a long-term, evolving condition has raised a host of issues for both the public policy and clinical agenda.

Foremost among these issues is reimbursement. Despite evidence of the benefits of early CKD identification and intervention, the structure of the current health care system devotes most of its resources toward disease-based medical care focused on costly chronic care interventions. Per capita spending for health care in the United States is more than double that in most developed nations, yet the United States ranks among the lowest in health access and health outcomes.[80, 81] Indeed, CKD is a microcosm of one of the deepest problems confronting the U.S. health care system: how to move from a system focused almost exclusively on procedure-oriented treatment of chronic disease to one that strikes a reasonable balance between treatment and prevention.

But the larger societal issue for CKD also involves the recognition that medical science has advanced to the point at which nephrologists are now able to intervene at earlier stages of CKD and slow, stop, or even reverse progression of the disease, as well as improve outcomes for kidney-related and comorbid-related medical complications. Prevention is no longer a lofty aspiration, but an achievable clinical reality.

An example of this advancing clinical knowledge in early kidney disease is the recognition that the high prevalence and morbid nature of CV disease in the early stages of CKD provide an opportunity to address those modifiable risk factors. The common co-occurrence of select CV disease risk factors, including hypertension and diabetes, which mirror CKD risk factors, has led to the description of the metabolic syndrome (MetS) in anticipation of a unifying pathogenesis and clinical prediction of CV disease.[82] The World Health Association recognizes CKD (as proteinuria) as a MetS criterion, in contrast to the third report of the National Cholesterol Education Program, which does not.[83, 84] Thus, key U.S. clinical guidelines currently overlook the importance of CKD as an important evidence-based CV disease risk factor and miss an outstanding opportunity to reinforce the significance of CKD identification and intervention for PCPs.

Another issue is quality of care. Although ESRD care is nearly universally available, disparities in care exist.[85] Moreover, the absence of adequate reimbursement for earlier stages of CKD care has left already-vulnerable patients at greater risk regarding preparation for dialysis and kidney transplantation, which is compounded by greater malnutrition, anemia, and other treatable conditions.[86, 87, 88]

Policy Recommendations

Box 9.1 presents a set of policy and clinical recommendations about how to advance the treatment of CKD. These recommendations were developed by the authors to provide a blueprint for reengineering CKD in the United States. The recommendations are intended to address the major challenges for CKD clinics and practices, which were summarized in Chapter Two. In addition, we also offer recommendations in two other key areas: HIT and research.

Each area of recommendation can be summarized as follows:

- Appropriate reimbursement must be available to screen at-risk populations and enable ongoing care by physicians by identifying patients at risk for progression or premature CKD.
- Patient referral should involve negotiation between nephrologists and other specialists at the local clinic or practice level, as well as at the level of the pertinent professional societies.
- Screening for CKD by eGFR should be made obligatory by Medicare and state Medicaid agencies, and private insurers should be strongly encouraged to pay for such screening. Appropriate education should be provided to physicians about how to interpret the results, particularly emphasizing the pitfalls of eGFR in certain populations, including the elderly.[89]
- Education is critical. Both patients and providers should be educated about the prevalence of CKD, who is at risk, who should be treated, and which treatments are effective in slowing the progression of the disease and treating its complications.*
- CKD clinical practice should integrate the efforts of PCPs, cardiologists, endocrinologists, and nephrologists, along with nonphysician care providers, to optimize clinical outcomes. Coordinated care management relying on available best medical evidence should drive clinical decisions and practice.
- Available clinical practice guidelines need to be integrated into clinical practice, include those published by KDOQI and RPA.
- Consistent with current health reform efforts, a robust HIT system is essential to track and evaluate care across various delivery sites.
- Nephrologists and other providers should be held accountable for patient outcomes.
- Substantial investments in translational and health services research are needed to understand how to prevent CKD, treat it when it occurs, and carry out these activities effectively and efficiently.

---

* Unfortunately, the Medicare Improvements for Patients and Providers Act of 2008 (MIPPA) excludes dialysis facilities as sites where education can be provided.

Box 9.1: Recommendations for Improving Chronic Kidney Disease Care, 2010

Economic/Reimbursement

1. Provide adequate reimbursement for CKD care in a nephrologist's office, including adequate payment for nonphysician services (i.e., physician assistants, nurses, dietitians).
2. Eliminate financial disincentives for screening of CKD patients.
3. Adequately reimburse facility costs for CKD clinics.
4. Develop evaluation and management (E and M) reimbursement with appropriate severity-of-illness adjusters.
5. Direct federal, state, and local government funding to CKD in high-risk populations.
6. Create "empowerment zones" to facilitate access to CKD care for underserved patients wherever these zones already exist for other purposes.
7. Consider a prospective payment system to cover care for CKD stage 4 and 5 patients.

Patient Referral

1. Facilitate transparent interaction between nephrologists and non-nephrologists.
2. Modify the standard of care for non-nephrologists to include appropriate, early referral to a nephrologist.
3. Require the Joint Commission on the Accreditation of Healthcare Organizations (JCAHO) to include appropriate referral to a nephrologist for any hospitalized patient with a discharge diagnosis of CKD as a requirement for hospital certification.

Screening

1. Require all government-sponsored health care entities to report eGFR on any patient who has a serum creatinine ordered.
2. Encourage all health insurers and health plans to reimburse for eGFR.
3. Have eGFR added as a Healthcare Effectiveness Data and Information Set (HEDIS) measure for health plans for relevant at-risk groups.

Education

1. Utilize all appropriate sites for education, including dialysis facilities, especially for approved education of stage 4 CKD patients.
2. Extend patient education to stage 3 CKD patients.
3. Reimburse the costs of patient education, even at early stages.
4. Emphasize in teaching materials for patients and physicians that the progression of CKD can be slowed even in advanced stages.
5. Develop culturally sensitive patient educational materials.
6. Encourage partnerships with community organizations and institutions serving vulnerable populations.
7. Develop end-of-life education for patients with CKD and reimburse the costs of development and implementation.

Box 9.1—Continued

Practice Organization

1. Integrate care across venues and domains of care.
2. Where feasible and reimbursed, provide CKD care in a CKD clinic with a multi-disciplinary team.
3. Organize CKD clinics to provide holistic care for patients with CKD.
4. Target care-coordination programs to high-risk and vulnerable populations.
5. Provide culturally competent care and language-concordant providers and staff.

Use of Clinical Practice Guidelines

1. Integrate available evidence-based CPGs into clinical practice, including NKF KDOQI and RPA CPGs.
2. Use and track performance measures based on CPGs to monitor and guide quality of care for CKD patients.

Health Information Technology

1. Use electronic health records (EHRs) for ongoing care of CKD patients.
2. Use EHRs to drive clinical practice, including the collection and analysis of data.

Nephrologist Accountability

1. Ensure that the discipline of nephrology emphasizes the commitment to improve and participate in CKD care prior to initiation of dialysis.
2. Ensure that nephrologists are accessible and available to nonphysician colleagues to ensure coordinated, transparent care of CKD patients.
3. Ensure that nephrologists are accountable for clinical outcomes in CKD patients and embrace a culture of accountability.

Research

1. Increase basic research on the causes and prevention of CKD.
2. Focus clinical research on the most effective means of slowing the progression of CKD.
3. Enhance health services research to better understand the most effective and efficient approaches to caring for patients with CKD.
4. Include minorities (e.g., women and disadvantaged groups) as appropriate in all research approaches, to better understand and to reduce CKD disparities in these groups.

Concluding Thoughts

The crisis of nephrology lies in an unresolved tension between the specialty's increasing ability to do the right thing clinically (by providing effective preventive care and even reversing the disease's progress) and the persistent realities of major barriers to doing so, including inadequate reimbursement, weak working relations between nephrology and other specialties, organizational impediments, ineffective clinical procedures, and a lack of HIT systems. The identification and treatment of the risk factors and complications of kidney disease per se, along with associated comorbid conditions, is increasingly understood. However, the lack of public policies makes the application of this body of evidence difficult to implement, especially among uninsured or underinsured populations.

Existing Medicare experience offers several ways in which our findings and recommendations can affect CKD disparities. First, the Medicare ESRD program provides a policy framework that can be extended to CKD relatively easily and need not be created *de novo*. Second, sufficient clinical knowledge of both ESRD and CKD exists on which to base informed policy actions. Finally, we know from nearly four decades of ESRD experience that extending Medicare entitlement to include CKD will improve access to care, will reduce disparities, and will require clinicians to deal with these disparities in the patients they encounter. For example, many of the early studies uncovering as well as showing improvement in racial disparities have been described in the Medicare population.[90, 91, 92, 93] To the extent that our observations identify models of improved access to CKD care for all individuals as well as efforts targeted on minority populations, this work may help eliminate disparities in kidney disease outcomes. Action on CKD policy will equip clinicians with the basic tools to respond to such factors.

Interview Template

Date:
Interview with:
Organization:
Contact information:
Interviewer: Dick Rettig

Notes:

Questions about Chronic Kidney Disease and CKD disparities among minority populations:

1. How do you rank the importance of early stage (Stage 1 or 2) interventions versus late stage (Stage 3 or 4) interventions for Chronic Kidney Disease (CKD) in slowing progression to End-Stage Renal Disease (ESRD)?
2. How is CKD care organized in your own clinical practice (e.g. CKD clinic, nurse practitioner)?
3. What problems or challenges have you encountered in trying to treat CKD patients?
4. What are the most common causes of CKD in your practice?
5. What are the primary referral sources of CKD in your practice?
6. What differences in CKD incidence and prevalence have you seen among minority populations when compared to non-minority patients?
7. In your practice do you think patients are referred too early or too late?
   a. Are there groups of patients that you think fare worse in CKD or present at more advanced stages (e.g., impoverished patients, geographically isolated patients, minority patients, or those who don't speak English)?
   b. What percent of your practice is from these groups?
8. How have you responded to such differences?
9. If CKD treatment is to be provided to all (i.e., as extensively as ESRD treatment currently is), what needs to be done?
   a. In your local practice?
   b. In your local community?
   c. In relation to other medical specialties?
   d. In relation to private health insurers?
   e. In relation to state Medicaid programs?
   f. In relation to Congress, CMS and the Medicare ESRD program?

10. If CKD disparities between minority and non-minority populations are to be sharply reduced, what needs to be done?
    a. In your local practice?
    b. In your local community?
    c. In relation to other medical specialties?
    d. In relation to private health insurers?
    e. In relation to state Medicaid programs?
    f. In relation to Congress, CMS and the Medicare ESRD program?
11. What other observations would you make about CKD, especially as it is manifest in minority populations?
12. Do you have any additional comments?

Endnotes

[1] Clinical Practice Guidelines for Chronic Kidney Disease: Evaluation, classification, and stratification. *American Journal of Kidney Disease*. 2002;39:2 (Suppl.1) [hereafter CKD guidelines].

[2] U.S. Renal Data System, *USRDS 2008 Annual Data Report: Atlas of Chronic Kidney Disease and End-Stage Renal Disease in the United States*, National Institutes of Health, National Institute of Diabetes and Digestive and Kidney Diseases, Bethesda, MD, 2008.

[3] Foley RN, Murray AM, Li S, Herzog CA, McBean AM, Eggers PW, Collins AJ. Chronic kidney disease and the risk for cardiovascular disease, renal replacement, and death in the United States Medicare population, 1998 to 1999. *J Am Soc Nephrol*. 2005;16:489–495.

[4] Go AS, Chertow GM, Fan D, McCulloch CE, Hsu CY. Chronic kidney disease and the risks of death, cardiovascular events, and hospitalization. *N Engl J Med*. 2004;351:1296–1305.

[5] U.S. Renal Data System. U.S. Department of Health and Human Services, Public Health Service, National Institutes of Health, Bethesda, MD, 2006.

[6] U.S. Renal Data System. *USRDS 2008 Annual Data Report*, Vol. 3, Table B1, 31.

[7] U.S. Renal Data System, *USRDS 2008 Annual Data Report: Atlas of Chronic Kidney Disease and End-Stage Renal Disease in the United States*, National Institutes of Health, National Institute of Diabetes and Digestive and Kidney Diseases, Bethesda, MD, 2008, Vol. 2;176–186.

[8] Bryan FA. Research Triangle Institute. The National Dialysis Registry: Fourth Annual Report: July 1, 1971–June 30, 1972.

[9] The 13th Report of the Human Renal Transplant Registry. *Transplantation Proceedings*. 1977;9:1,9–26.

[10] Martins D, Tareen N, Norris KC. The epidemiology of end-stage renal disease among African Americans. *Am J Med Sci*. 2002 Feb;323(2):65–71.

[11] Mitka M. Report notes increase in kidney disease. *JAMA*. 2008 Dec 3;300(21):2473–2474.

[12] U.S. Renal Data System. *USRDS 2008 Annual Data Report*, Vol. 2, Atlas of End-Stage Renal Disease, 62.

[13] U.S. Renal Data System. *USRDS 2008 Annual Data Report*, Section D, Treatment Modalities, 80.

[14] U.S. Renal Data System. *USRDS 2008 Annual Data Report*, Vol. 3, 7 (incidence) and 31 (prevalence).

[15] Murray CJ, Kulkarni SC, Michaud C, Tomijima N, Bulzacchelli MT, Iandiorio TJ, Ezzati M. Eight Americas: Investigating mortality disparities across races, counties, and race-counties in the United States. *PLoS Med*. 2006 Sep;3(9):e260.

[16] Norris KC, Agodoa LY. Unraveling the racial disparities associated with kidney disease. *Kidney Int*. 2005;68:914–924.

[17] Schroeder S. Shattuck Lecture: We can do better—improving the health of the American people. *N Engl J Med*. 2007;357:1221–1228.

[18]   Lurie N, Jung M, Lavizzo-Mourey R. *Health Aff* (Millwood). 2005 Mar-Apr;24(2):354–364.

[19]   Groman R, Ginsburg J. American College of Physicians. *Ann Intern Med*. 2004 Aug 3;141(3):226–232.

[20]   Washington DL, Bowles J, Saha S, Horowitz CR, Moody-Ayers S, Brown AF, Stone VE, Cooper LA. Writing group for the Society of General Internal Medicine, Disparities in Health Task Force. *J Gen Intern Med*. 2008 May;23(5):685–691. Epub 2008 Jan 15.

[21]   Lurie N, Fremont A, Somers SA, Coltin K, Gelzer A, Johnson R, Rawlins W, Ting G, Wong W, Zimmerman D. The National Health Plan Collaborative to Reduce Disparities and Improve Quality. *Jt Comm J Qual Patient Saf*. 2008 May;34(5):256–265.

[22]   Powe NR, Melamed ML. Racial disparities in the optimal delivery of chronic kidney disease care. *Med Clin N Am*. 2005;89:475–488.

[23]   Seghal AR. Impact of quality improvement efforts on race and sex disparities in hemodialysis. *JAMA*. 2003;289:996–1000.

[24]   Ayanian JZ, Cleary PD, Weissman JS, Epstein AM. The effect of patients' preferences on racial differences in access to renal transplantation. *N Engl J Med*. 1999; 341:1661–1669.

[25]   CKD guidelines.

[26]   Glassock RJ, Winearls C. Screening for CKD with eGFR: Doubts and dangers. *Clin J Am Soc Nephrol*. 2008 Sep;3(5):1563–1568.

[27]   Jungers P. Late referral: Loss of chance for the patient, loss of money for society. *Nephrol Dial Trans*. 2002;17:371–375.

[28]   Khan SS, et al. Does Nephrology care influence patient survival after initiation of dialysis? *Kid Int*. 2005;67(3):1038–1046.

[29]   Hayashi R, E Huang E, Nissenson AR. Vascular access for hemodialysis. *Nature Clin Pract Nephrol*. 2006;2(9)504–513.

[30]   *Fistula First Breakthrough Initiative Special Project Annual Report*; 2007. As of May 10, 2009: http://www.fistulafirst.org/pdfs/2007_Fistula_First_Annual_Report.pdf

[31]   Balamuthusamy S, Srinivasan L, Verma M, Adigopula S, Jalandara N, Hathiwala S, Smith E. Renin angiotensin system blockade and cardiovascular outcomes in patients with chronic kidney disease and proteinuria: A meta-analysis. *Am Heart J*. 2008 May;155(5):791–805.

[32]   KDOQI Clinical Practice Guidelines on Hypertension and Antihypertensive Agents in Chronic Kidney Disease: Executive summary. *Am J Kid Dis*. 2004;42(Suppl 1):16–33.

[33]   National Kidney Foundation. KDOQI clinical practice guidelines and clinical practice recommendations for diabetes and chronic kidney disease. *Am J Kid Dis*. 2007 Feb;49(2 Suppl 2):S12–154.

[34]   Rettig RA, interview with Andrew Levey, December 19, 2006.

[35]   National Kidney Foundation. KDOQI Clinical Practice Guidelines for Chronic Kidney Disease: Evaluation, classification, and stratification. *Am J Kid Dis*. 2002;39(Suppl 1):S1–S266.

[36]   Parker TF, Blantz R, Hostetter T, Himmelfarb J, Kliger A, Lazarus M, Nissenson AR, Pereira B, Weiss J. The Chronic Kidney Disease Initiative. *J Am Soc Nephrol*. 2004;15:708–716.

[37]   Parker TF, Blantz R, Hostetter T, Himmelfarb J, Kliger A, Lazarus M, Nissenson AR, Pereira B, Weiss J. The Chronic Kidney Disease Initiative. *J Am Soc Nephrol*. 2004;15(3):708–716.

[38]   Rettig RA, Levinsky NG, eds. *Kidney Failure and the Federal Government*, Washington, D.C.: National Academy Press; 1991.

[39] Vargas RB, Ryan GW, Jackson CA, Rodriguez R, Freeman HP. Characteristics of the original patient navigation programs to reduce disparities in the diagnosis and treatment of breast cancer. *Cancer.* 2008 Jul 15;113(2):426–433.

[40] Vargas RB, Mangione CM, Asch S, Keesey J, Rosen M, Schonlau M, Keeler EB. Can a chronic care model collaborative reduce heart disease risk in patients with diabetes? *J Gen Intern Med.* 2007 Feb;22(2):215–222.

[41] Vargas RB, Jones L, Terry C, Nicholas SB, Kopple J, Forge N, Griffin A, Louis M, Barba L, Small L, Norris KC. Building Bridges to Optimum Health World Kidney Day Los Angeles 2007 Collaborative. Community-partnered approaches to enhance chronic kidney disease awareness, prevention, and early intervention. *Adv Chronic Kidney Dis.* 2008 Apr;15(2):153–161.

[42] Rettig RA, Norris K, Nissenson AR. Chronic kidney disease in the United States: A policy imperative. *Clin J Am Soc Nephrol.* 2008;3:1902–1910.

[43] Ghossein C, Serrano A, Rammohan M, Batlle D. The role of comprehensive renal clinic in chronic kidney disease stabilization and management: The Northwestern experience. *Seminars in Nephrology.* 2002;22:526–532.

[44] Interview with James Paparello, M.D., May 2, 2007.

[45] Interview with Cybele Ghossein, M.D., May 2, 2007.

[46] Interview with Daniel Batlle, M.D., May 2, 2007.

[47] Serrano A, Huang J, Ghossein C, Nishi L, Gangavathi A, Madhan V, Ramadug P, Ahya SN, Paparell J, Khosla N, Schlueter W, Batlle D. Stabilization of glomerular filtration rate in advanced chronic kidney disease: A two-year follow-up of a cohort of chronic kidney disease patients stages 4 and 5. *Adv Chronic Kidney Dis.* 2007;14:109.

[48] Batlle interview, 2007.

[49] Serrano A, Huang J, Nishi L, Chilakapati R, Ghossein C, Paparello J, Ahya S, Khosla N, Rosa R, Weitzel M, Batlle D. *Four-year Follow-Up of a Cohort of Patients with Advanced CKD Management in an Academic CKD Clinic: Grounds for Optimism.* National Kidney Foundation, Orlando, 2007.

[50] Telephone interview with Daniel Batlle, M.D., May 9, 2006.

[51] Telephone interview with Batlle, 2006.

[52] Batlle interview, 2007.

[53] Batlle interview, 2007.

[54] Batlle D, Ramadugu P, Soler MJ. Progress in retarding the progression of advanced chronic kidney disease: Grounds for optimism. *Kidney Int.* 2006;70:S40–44.

[55] Ghossein et al., 527.

[56] Ghossein et al., 528.

[57] Ghossein interview.

[58] Ghossein interview.

[59] Serrano et al.

[60] Serrano et al., 108.

[61] Spangers B, et al. Late referral of patients with chronic kidney disease: No time to waste. *Mayo Clin Proc.* 2006 Nov;81(11):1487–1494.

[62] Crawford PW. Changing trends in referral source of ESRD patients in a nephrology practice between 1995 and 2005. Poster presentation. National Kidney Foundation Annual Clinical Meeting, spring 2006.

[63] Crawford PW, Roberts K. Anemia management in chronic kidney disease: Primary care physicians contrasted with nephrologists. Poster presentation. National Kidney Foundation Annual Clinical Meeting, spring 2006.

[64] Crawford PW, Roberts K. Anemia management in chronic kidney disease: Primary care physicians contrasted with nephrologists. Poster presentation. National Kidney Foundation Annual Clinical Meeting, spring 2006.

[65] Nissenson, A, et al. Opportunities for improving care of patients with chronic renal insufficiency: Current practice patterns. *JASN.* 12(8):1713–1720.

[66] Hemmelgarn, et al. Progressive kidney dysfunction in the elderly. *Kidney Int.* 2005;69:2155–2161.

[67] Chan, M., et al. Outcomes in patients with CKD referred late to nephrologists: A meta-analysis. *Am J Med.* 2007;120,1063–1070.

[68] Patwardhan, M, et al. Non-nephrologist and nephrologist perspectives on implementation of a CKD guideline. *JHQ.* 29(6):W6-3–W6-17.

[69] Renal Physicians Association. *The Advanced CKD Management Toolkit: Improving Management and Care of Advanced CKD Patients*; 2004. Rockville, MD.

[70] Coresh, et al. Prevalence of chronic kidney disease in the United States. *JAMA.* 2007 Nov 7;298:2038–2047.

[71] National Kidney Foundation: KDOQI Clinical Practice Guidelines for Chronic Kidney Disease: Evaluation, classification, and stratification. *Am J Kidney Dis.* 2002;39(2 Suppl 2):S1–S246.

[72] Renal Physicians Association: Appropriate Patient Preparation for Renal Replacement Therapy. Renal Physicians Association Clinical Practice Guideline #3. Rockville, MD, October 2002.

[73] Patwardhan, et al. Advanced CKD practice patterns among nephrologists and non-nephrologists: A database analysis. *CJASN.* 2007 Mar;2:277–283.

[74] McMurray SD, Johnson G, Davis S, McDougall K. Diabetes education and care management significantly improve patient outcomes in the dialysis unit. *Am J Kidney Dis.* 2002 Sept;40(3):566–575.

[75] Duru OK, Vargas RB, Kermah D, Nissenson AR, Norris KC. High prevalence of stage 3 chronic kidney disease in older adults despite normal serum creatinine. *J Gen Intern Med.* 2009 Jan;24(1):86–92.

[76] McMurray SD, and Howell AL. Disease management of chronic kidney disease improves patient management and outcomes. Poster presentation at American Society of Nephrology annual meeting, 2004.

[77] Murray and Howell.

[78] Duru OK, Vargas RB, Kermah D, Nissenson AR, Norris KC. High prevalence of stage 3 chronic kidney disease in older adults despite normal serum creatinine. *J Gen Intern Med.* 2009 Jan;24(1):86–92.

[79] Jungers, et al. *Kidney Int Suppl.* 1993 Jun;41:S170–S173.

[80] OECD Health Data 2007: How Does the United States Compare (Organization for Economic Cooperation and Development, 2007). As of April 5, 2010: http://www.oecd.org/dataoecd/46/2/38980580.pdf

[81] Davis K et al. *Mirror, Mirror on the Wall: An International Update on the Comparative Performance of American Health Care* (The Commonwealth Fund, 2007). As of April 5, 2010: http://www.commonwealthfund.org/usr_doc/1027_Davis_mirror_mirror_international_update_final.pdf?section=4039

[82] Isomaa B, Almgren P, Tuomi T, et al. Cardiovascular morbidity and mortality associated with the metabolic syndrome. *Diabetes Care.* 2001;24:683–689.

[83] Alberti KG, Zimmer PZ. Definition, diagnosis and classification of Diabetes Mellitus and its complications: Diagnosis and classification of Diabetes Mellitus provisional report of a WHO consultation. *Diabet Med.* 1998;15:539–553.

[84] Third Report of the National Cholesterol Education Program (NCEP) Expert Panel on Detection, Evaluation, and Treatment of High Blood Cholesterol in Adults (Adult Treatment Panel III) final report. Circulation 2002;106:3143–3421.

[85] Sehgal AR. Impact of quality improvement efforts on race and sex disparities in hemodialysis. *JAMA.* 2003;289(8):996–1000.

[86] Powe NR. To have and not to have: Health and health care disparities in chronic kidney disease. *Kidney Int.* 2003;64(2):763–772.

[87] Kinchen KS, Sadler J, Fink, et al. The timing of specialist evaluation in chronic kidney disease and mortality. *Ann Intern Med.* 2002;137(6):479–486.

[88] Ayanian JZ, Cleary PD, Weissman JS, et al. The effect of patients' preferences on racial differences in access to renal transplantation. *N Eng J Med.* 1999;341(22):1661–1669.

[89] Glassock RJ. Estimated glomerular filtration rate: Time for a performance review? *Kidney Int.* 2009;75:1001–1003.

[90] Wallace SP, Villa VM, Enriquez-Haass V, Mendez CA. Access is better for racial/ethnic elderly in Medicare HMOs—but disparities persist. Policy Brief, UCLA Cent Health Policy Res. 2001 May.

[91] Schneider EC, Zaslavsky AM, Epstein AM. Racial disparities in the quality of care for enrollees in medicare managed care. *JAMA.* 2002 Mar 13;287(10):1288–1294.

[92] Gornick ME, Eggers PW, Reilly TW, Mentnech RM, Fitterman LK, Kucken LE, Vladeck BC. Effects of race and income on mortality and use of services among Medicare beneficiaries. *N Engl J Med.* 1996 Sep 12;335(11):791–799.

[93] Ayanian JZ, Cleary PD, Weissman JS, Epstein AM. The effect of patients' preferences on racial differences in access to renal transplantation. *N Engl J Med.* 1999 Nov 25;341(22):1661–1669.